# GLUTEN FREE LIFE STYLE

## a health guide, shopping & home tips, 66 easy recipes

### by JOHN CHATHAM

# TABLE OF CONTENTS

# INTRODUCTION AND OVERVIEW

Gluten-free diets are not just the latest fad. Ever-increasing numbers of people are choosing to embrace gluten-free diets as awareness of celiac disease, wheat allergies and gluten intolerance grows. Whether you have decided to live gluten-free by necessity or by choice, following a gluten-free diet is a challenge. It is a lifestyle change that requires diligence, creativity and a commitment that will help you get past the daily hurdles.

*The Gluten-Free Lifestyle* is designed to help you make the transition to a gluten-free lifestyle with less confusion and more delicious recipes. I'll explain what gluten is, the different health issues people may have with gluten, and how to live without it and still enjoy great food.

It's important that you make your gluten-free decision an informed one. If you feel your body reacts badly to gluten or to wheat products, it is essential to be tested for celiac disease before you cut gluten from your diet. This test diagnoses the disease by looking for specific antibodies—antibodies that will not be present after you are no longer eating gluten. That's why you must take the test before you change your diet.

**DID YOU KNOW?** *According to a recent article in WebMD, "If you think you might have celiac disease, the biggest mistake is to begin a diet without being tested," says Stefano Guandalini, MD, director of the University of Chicago Celiac Disease Center.*

*"The test really has to be done before [quitting gluten]. If you don't do the test and begin the diet, your antibodies slowly but progressively decrease and become normal within three to six months."*

It is essential to understand the exact reason why your body doesn't tolerate gluten, because there are important differences between celiac disease, wheat allergy and gluten sensitivity. It's also the only way you'll know if other family members are affected, since celiac disease tends to be inherited. Once you know why your health is affected by eating gluten or wheat, you'll know how seriously you need to take going gluten-free, whether your problem is all types of gluten or just wheat, and whether deviating from the gluten-free diet is a matter of choice or a matter of safety.

Gluten is a compound protein that, along with starch, is stored in the endosperm of certain grassy grains, such as wheat, barley and rye. The endosperm is the part of a seed that stores food for the developing plant embryo. The presence of gluten in flour is what gives dough its elasticity, helps it rise and imparts a chewy texture to foods like bread.

Gluten can be removed from dough by rinsing the unrisen dough in water. This separated gluten is used as a stabilizer in many products that don't ordinarily contain flour, and is also used to add protein to foods that are naturally low in protein. This is what is known as "hidden gluten," since most people are unaware of the gluten content in those foods and the FDA doesn't require it to be included in ingredient labels.

When you make a decision to eat a gluten-free diet, it suddenly seems that gluten is in everything—and it is in a great deal of things you might not expect. It can be difficult at first to weed out all of foods you're used to eating but can no longer have.

Fortunately, there are plenty of ways to enjoy some of your favorite foods by using recipes that take traditional favorites and make them without wheat, barley, rye or oats. I've included many wonderful recipes in the cookbook section of this book, and even a bonus selection of gluten-free treats you may have thought you'd have to do without, such as fudgy brownies, pizza and even French bread.

# CELIAC DISEASE, WHEAT ALLERGY AND GLUTEN SENSITIVITY

The reported number of patients diagnosed with some form of poor reaction to gluten is on the rise in Western countries. The reason for this is not fully understood. Some blame it on the high amounts of processed foods, breads and baked goods in the Western diet. Another theory is that we are not exposed to enough antigens during childhood as our immune systems are developing. Because of this, our immune systems see gluten as an interloper or allergen.

There are three main types of diagnoses related to gluten reactions: celiac disease, wheat allergy and gluten sensitivity. Since they share many symptoms, it's important to get a correct diagnosis from your doctor, because a self-diagnosis based on your symptoms stands a decent chance of being incorrect and can lead to the wrong corrective action.

## Celiac Disease

Celiac disease is considered the most serious of the three types of gluten reactions, and is often misdiagnosed as irritable bowel syndrome or a food intolerance such as wheat allergy. Often, it is only when treatment for these issues doesn't alleviate symptoms that doctors begin looking at celiac disease as a possibility.

If celiac disease is suspected, a doctor will order blood tests to detect and measure two types of antibodies: IgAtTG (Immunoglobulin A [IgA] anti-tissue transglutaminase [tTG] antibody) and IgAEMA (Immunoglobulin A [IgA] antiendomysial antibody [EMA]). If these antibodies are detected, doctors often confirm the diagnosis of celiac disease with a biopsy of the small intestine conducted during an endoscopy. An endoscopy is performed by guiding a small scope (called an endoscope) into the small intestine via the throat.

The small intestine is lined with microscopic projections that look a bit like sea anemone, called villi. The job of the villi is to absorb vitamins, fats and other nutrients from foods as they pass through the small intestine. What's left is waste and moves on to the large intestine to be eliminated.

In a person with celiac disease, the villi flatten out and the lining of the small intestine becomes swollen or inflamed. This decreases the absorption of nutrients and can result in stunted growth, anemia, osteoporosis and malnutrition. This inability to absorb nutrients is often what alerts doctors to celiac disease in children, as they fail to grow and gain weight at a normal rate.

One of the reasons celiac disease is underdiagnosed is that it produces a wide array of symptoms that can vary in incidence and severity. They include:

- Gas
- Abdominal swelling
- Bloating
- Constipation
- Diarrhea
- Fatty stools
- Weight loss despite normal appetite

- Anemia
- Frequent headaches
- Nausea
- Vomiting
- Fatigue

Because of the decreased absorption of nutrients, celiac disease can also result in depression, frequent respiratory infections, delayed puberty, trouble with memory or concentration, and irritability.

The treatment for celiac disease is a gluten-free diet, often accompanied by vitamin supplementation to correct common deficiencies. Many people with celiac disease tend to be deficient in fat-soluble vitamins such as A, D, K and E. That's because in people with the disease, fat is poorly absorbed from the intestines. And when fat is not absorbed, the vitamins that dissolve in it are also not absorbed. Frequently, levels of calcium, iron, magnesium, zinc, folate, selenium and copper are also low, for the same reason, and need to be supplemented.

### Lactose Intolerance and Celiac Disease

Some people diagnosed with celiac disease also find that they are lactose intolerant. This is because of the damage done to the villi in the small intestine. The cells lining the small intestine produce an enzyme called lactase. Lactase is necessary for digesting lactose, which is the sugar that occurs naturally in milk and milk products. The damage that causes celiac disease results in both a deficiency of lactase and the villi's inability to catch and break down lactose molecules.

If you've just been diagnosed with celiac disease, ask your doctor about testing you for lactose intolerance as well. Don't be discouraged about having to give up another food group. In many cases, the lactose intolerance is only temporary. In most cases, the villi are able to repair themselves within six months to a year after going gluten-free. However, lactose intolerance and its symptoms can continue for some time after you go on a gluten-free diet; sometimes for as long as two years.

After you have been gluten-free for a year, ask your doctor to retest you for lactose intolerance. Your small intestine and villi may be healthy enough to produce sufficient lactase by this time.

Until then, you can substitute almond milk, soy milk or rice milk for drinking, cooking and lightening your coffee. You can even find cheese, yogurt and ice cream made from these dairy alternatives.

## Wheat Allergy

People with a wheat allergy may initially suspect they have celiac disease. This is an understandable assumption, since the two problems share many common symptoms and those symptoms are triggered by eating many of the same foods. Only proper testing can correctly identify the problem. The symptoms of a wheat allergy vary in intensity, based largely on the amount of wheat eaten. They include:

- Swelling, itching or irritation of the mouth or throat
- Hives, itchy rash or swelling of the skin
- Nasal congestion
- Itchy, watery eyes
- Difficulty breathing
- Cramps, nausea or vomiting
- Diarrhea
- Anaphylaxis (swelling of the throat, difficulty breathing)

In a person with wheat allergy, the allergen is the wheat itself, not the gluten. This means people with a wheat allergy can't eat foods containing wheat and wheat flour, but, unlike people with celiac disease, they can safely eat foods made with barley, rye and oats. Wheat allergy is one of the most common food allergies found in children.

Some people with a wheat allergy choose to go on a gluten-free diet because it seems simpler and they feel it may be a healthier diet overall.

## Gluten Sensitivity

Gluten sensitivity has only recently been recognized as a condition separate from celiac disease. Although the cause of gluten sensitivity is still being intensely researched, the medical community now agrees that it is a separate disorder.

There is no specific diagnostic test for gluten sensitivity. Your doctor will generally use your medical history and a physical examination, combined with your own reporting of symptoms you experience when eating products made with or containing gluten. Doctors often rule out celiac disease first. Even if the key diagnostic antibodies are present, the villi and small intestine will not show the damage that occurs in people with celiac disease.

The symptoms of gluten sensitivity are often the same as those of celiac disease, although they may differ in severity or frequency. The most common symptoms include:

- Gastrointestinal distress (particularly gas, bloating and nausea)
- Frequent headaches
- Fatigue

Commonly, doctors advise a gluten-free diet for those with gluten sensitivity, although these patients will probably not require additional vitamin supplements, since they suffer some of the same reactions to gluten but not the villi damage that inhibits nutrient absorption.

Whether you've chosen to adopt a gluten-free diet because of celiac disease, wheat allergy or gluten sensitivity, you can expect to feel a great deal better once you've been on a gluten-free diet for a short time. If you don't see a marked improvement in symptoms, it's extremely important to see your doctor to rule out any other conditions, such as Crohn's disease or irritable bowel syndrome.

# ( 2 )

# WERE OUR BODIES DESIGNED TO EAT GLUTEN?

The rising number of people diagnosed with celiac disease and gluten sensitivity has attracted more attention to the theory that our bodies are not genetically designed to eat grains. This theory is what has led to the popularity of the Paleolithic, Paleo or Stone Age diets.

There are some scientific studies that support this theory. It's true that until about 10,000 years ago, grains were not cultivated and so were not a part of the daily human diet. It's also true that people in pre-agricultural times did not seem to have suffered from various metabolic and digestive disorders that have been attributed to eating grains and processed foods such as breads, cereals, pastries and other modern favorites. The rate of metabolic syndrome, type 2 diabetes, obesity and other such disorders has risen dramatically in the past few decades, and many nutritionists and researchers blame the fact that processed grains make up a growing proportion of the typical daily diet.

Researchers and nutritionists who have recommended removing grains and legumes from our diets suggest that our bodies have not had enough time to adapt genetically to absorbing and processing grains. Since gluten comes from grains, it may follow that we're not genetically adapted to eating it, either.

**DID YOU KNOW?** *For 2.5 million years, humans ate no wheat, rice, corn, barley or oats. We have only been consuming these foods for about 10,000 years. In other words, for 99.6 percent of our history, we were not grain-eaters.*

The jury is still out on whether eating grains is bad for our health. But quite a few people have chosen to follow diets like the Paleo diet, which is a gluten-free diet that is also very high in protein. Many people following the Paleo diet report better digestive health, more energy and less inflammation.

Scientists can't confidently say that all grains are bad for your health. They do know that wheat, barley, rye and possibly oats are dangerous for those with celiac disease and gluten sensitivity, and that wheat and wheat products are a health threat to those with a wheat allergy.

# 3

## IS A GLUTEN-FREE DIET HEALTHY FOR EVERYONE?

O bviously, a gluten-free diet is essential for those who have been diagnosed with either celiac disease or gluten sensitivity. It's also a simple option for those who have a wheat allergy, as it takes much of the guesswork and label-reading out of the equation. But is going gluten-free beneficial to the rest of us? The answer is maybe.

### Eliminating or Limiting Processed Foods Is Always a Good Idea

Eliminating or greatly reducing prepared or convenience foods from your diet is always a good thing. Many of these foods are high in fats, sugar and other ingredients that you simply don't need in a healthy diet—in any form. Empty calories (calories with little nutrition) come from heavily processed foods and snacks such as cookies, cakes, crackers, pasta, sugary cereals, buns and rolls. By not eating them, we can make our diets significantly healthier and more nutritious.

## Eliminating Grains May Very Well Be a Good Idea

Researchers and scientists agree that humans have only been eating grains for less than 1 percent of our history as a species. There's still a good deal of debate about whether that fact has any significance when it comes to health and nutrition, but many well-respected nutritionists believe it does. Many followers of diets such as the Paleo diet agree, and they report feeling much better overall, with fewer digestive issues and headaches, and an increase in energy.

If you're going gluten-free because you think it might be healthier, or if you have a wheat allergy and are going gluten-free altogether, you'll likely be reducing the unhealthy fats, sugars and preservatives that often come with flour-based foods.

**DID YOU KNOW?** *If your child has been diagnosed with celiac disease or gluten sensitivity, you have no option but to put them on a gluten-free diet. As long as your children are getting plenty of protein, fats, healthy carbohydrates and fiber from plant foods, they'll be getting a balanced diet that may even be healthier than one that includes gluten.*

# LOSING WEIGHT ON A GLUTEN-FREE DIET

A gluten-free diet is not necessarily a weight-loss diet. In fact, if you're not careful, you could actually gain weight once you go gluten-free. It is possible to lose weight while on a gluten-free diet, but you will need to follow some guidelines.

## Beware of Hidden Fat and Sugar

Ready-to-eat gluten-free products can be useful for those who choose to live gluten-free, but it is important to read food labels carefully to see exactly what you're eating. Gluten-free processed foods, such as cookies, crackers, breads, cereals and desserts, present some of the same problems that low-fat and nonfat products did when they became popular. Many people felt cheated or tricked when they found out that some of these products had more sugar and calories than the full-fat versions. Similarly, many gluten-free processed foods contain a great deal of both sugar and fat to enhance taste and improve texture.

## Watch Out for Overeating

It's easy to unintentionally eat too much of foods that we perceive as being healthy. You may have run into this problem when "100-calorie" snack packets hit the shelves, or when you found out that healthy smoothies were packed with calories and needed to be eaten as a treat rather than a daily staple. Many of us believe more is better and eat more in general. Some studies have shown that overeating alone can account for the obesity epidemic in America.

## Be Sure to Eat Frequently

Skipping meals lowers your blood sugar and raises your insulin levels. This creates cravings for quick-fix carbohydrates, which you're probably used to getting from things like cereal, bread, fruit and grain bars, cookies and other foods made from the easily absorbed carbohydrates contained in grains.

If you skip meals, you'll be setting yourself up for either eating something that will hurt you (if you have celiac disease or gluten sensitivity), or eating something that's just not good for you—and certainly not good for weight loss, like a soda or candy bar.

By eating at least every two hours or so, you can avoid many of these carbohydrate cravings and increase your chances of losing weight on a gluten-free diet.

## Get Plenty of Fiber

If you've been getting most of your fiber from healthy, whole-grain cereals and breads, you're going to need to increase your plant fiber intake. Overall, plant fiber has been shown to be a healthier fiber choice than the fiber from grains.

Be sure to eat plenty of the most fibrous fruits and vegetables, including apples, mangoes, papaya, broccoli, Brussels sprouts and celery. Plant foods contain soluble (dissolves in water) and insoluble (doesn't dissolve in water) fiber, and both are real powerhouses. As long as you eat a wide variety of fresh fruits and vegetables daily, you'll keep your fiber intake at a healthy level. If you're one of those people who have trouble getting enough fruits and veggies, consider adding psyllium husk to smoothies, shakes, baked goods and even scrambled eggs.

## Get Plenty of Protein

Breads, pasta and cereals make up a huge chunk of the daily calories most Americans eat. If you cut them from your diet and don't replace them with gluten-free options, you're likely to cut your calories way down, too.

If you find yourself feeling hungry frequently, take a look at your calorie intake and make sure you're eating enough. Protein will help you feel satisfied. Make sure you eat plenty of healthy protein, such as lean meats, fish, shellfish, eggs and dairy (if you can have it). You'll increase calories in a healthy way and the protein will make you feel full longer than the empty calories of fats or carbohydrates.

## Drink Plenty of Water

Dieters get tired of hearing about how they need to drink plenty of water, but water aids digestion, helps you feel full and even helps your body get rid of excess stored fat. Going gluten-free means changes to your digestive system—changes that will be helped along by getting adequate water (64 ounces a day—more if you work out or spend much time outdoors).

**DID YOU KNOW?** *Don't be fooled into thinking you need less water during the colder months. Your lungs absorb water as well as oxygen, and when the humidity is lower, so is your water intake through respiration. You'll also need to be sure to drink extra water if you're at a high altitude (more than 3,000 feet above sea level), if you fly or if you're under more than usual stress.*

Don't be discouraged or assume that your weight loss goals will have to be put on hold if you go on a gluten-free diet. As long as you follow these guidelines, eat sensibly and get plenty of exercise, you can lose weight on a gluten-free diet.

Later on, I'll provide you with some sample menus to help you plan your weight loss on a gluten-free diet.

# How to Transition to Gluten-Free

# REAL WORLD GLUTEN-FREE—HOW IT WORKS

Going on any diet requires some work. You have to plan, strategize, compromise and commit. When your diet is required medically, there's the added stress of knowing you can't just quit when you get bored or frustrated. But for any diet to be successful, you have to be able to stick with it. The best diets:

- Are as easy as possible to follow
- Provide plenty of nutrition and variety
- Give you ways to enjoy the foods you really love
- Are accessible and affordable for everyone
- Are convenient

That's what I've put together for you in these pages—a way to go gluten-free in the real world, no matter what your budget is, how busy you are, how much you love good food or what your family situation is. You can go on this diet if:

- You're a single person living alone, or the parent of several children
- You have plenty to spend on specialty groceries, or are on a tight food budget
- You are a gourmet, or don't really enjoy cooking

- You have hours to spend making homemade meals, or need menus that are fast and easy

Real world gluten-free living means being able to stick with your diet no matter how busy you are, or whether you're in a restaurant or your own home. It means you have to be able to feed yourself without going broke or feeling like your diet is a part-time job. It means knowing how to stick with your diet without feeling separate from everyone else.

## Knowing What You Can Eat and What You Cannot

This is the most important part of going gluten-free. A gluten-free diet isn't as simple as going vegetarian or even going on a raw-food diet. Gluten is in so many products and comes in so many forms that reading labels is essential. The lists of Allowed and Not Allowed Foods in this book are extensive, and I've arranged them in alphabetical order rather than food groups to make it easier for you to look up a specific (and often unfamiliar) ingredient when you're checking labels. Print out a copy to take to the stores with you, or to have handy when you're shopping online.

## Knowing How to Replace the Foods You Cannot Have

It's easy and very common to get discouraged and upset when you think you can never again have chocolate cake, a blueberry muffin or a hearty sandwich. Fortunately, going gluten-free in the real world means you can have your cake and eat it too. The recipe collection here includes gluten-free ways to enjoy many of your favorite foods, and the resources section includes links to thousands more. You'll be able to find plenty of gluten-free recipes for everything from pizza to pasta and brownies to cupcakes.

## Knowing How to Eat No Matter Where You Are

Most people don't have the option of going gluten-free in a bubble—nor would we want to. We eat in restaurants, at the homes of friends and on food-centered holidays. As you go through this book, you'll find tips and guidelines for eating safely when you're dining out, when you're at a party or when you are celebrating Thanksgiving and other special days with your loved ones.

You'll also find a section on making your home safe without alienating your family or yourself. I'll tell you what you need to know to cook both for yourself and for the rest of your household without worrying about cross-contamination, and how to prepare foods that everyone can eat without having to cook two separate meals.

## Have Plenty of Choices, No Matter How Busy You Are, How Little You Cook or How Tight Your Budget Is

Some of us love to cook and have plenty of time to spend doing it. Others are on very tight schedules or just don't enjoy spending much time in the kitchen. The recipe selection and the resources in this book will give you a wide array of foods that suit your needs and lifestyle. There are quick and easy meals you can throw together in a snap, as well as more involved recipes for those who love to bake homemade breads or fix meals from scratch.

The resources section will also point you to several retailers and websites where you can purchase packaged cereals, baked goods and other foods that are gluten-free. Don't worry—even if you don't have the time or desire to bake your own gluten-free cookies or breads, you won't have to go without.

Gluten-free packaged foods can be expensive, especially if you're also buying traditional versions for the rest of the family. If you're on a tight grocery budget, you can save a great deal of money by using the recipes here and many others to prepare your own gluten-free foods at home—at a fraction of the cost.

Going gluten-free isn't necessarily simple, and it definitely isn't without compromise. But going gluten-free in the real world can be delicious, affordable and easier than you think.

# 6

# HIDDEN GLUTEN—THE SURPRISING PLACES GLUTEN HIDES

There is a reason why I chose to present the Allowed and Not Allowed Foods Lists in alphabetical order. You're going to be reading a lot of labels, and many of those labels will contain unfamiliar ingredients.

Various groups are working with the FDA and food manufacturers to come up with better labeling to inform consumers about when gluten is present in a product. But until then, it's up to you to know what you're eating. Having an alphabetical list handy will help you immensely when you're doing your grocery shopping. However, you need to be aware that gluten is used in many nonfood products as well.

## Foods You Might Not Realize Have Gluten

As you'll see later in the Not Allowed Foods List, gluten is in a lot of food products that don't come to mind when you're thinking about wheat, barley, rye and their byproducts. For instance, many types of vinegar are made of malt, which is a barley product. Now you know to avoid malt vinegar, but many salad dressings, barbecue sauces and steak sauces will list vinegar on their ingredients list without telling you what kind of vinegar.

Many soy sauces contain gluten as well. Condiments are a tricky group overall. Many commercial mayonnaises use gluten as a binder and stabilizer. Some mustards contain gluten as well. Tomato sauces sometimes contain gluten, and tomato paste often does. These items can show up in commercial ketchups, spaghetti sauces and barbecue sauces. The problem is that only "tomato paste" is listed in the ingredients.

---

**DID YOU KNOW?** *Medications frequently contain gluten. Pills are often dusted with flour during the manufacturing process, and the oil in capsules may include gluten too. Check with your pharmacist to see if your medication is safe for you. If they are unsure, call the manufacturer. There are websites that list gluten-free medications, and I've included some of them in the resources section.*

---

Part of the issue with hidden gluten is that it can be used in the packaging or processing of a product, too, without it actually being considered an ingredient. For instance, some gums are dusted with wheat and other flours to keep them from being sticky. Candy bars may be made without gluten, but the conveyor belts on which they are processed are often dusted with wheat flour.

Yeast may be either grown or dried on wheat. Wheat is sometimes added to ice cream to prevent the formation of ice crystals. There may be wheat flour in your spices, too, particularly spice blends like Cajun or Italian seasonings. Crispy rice cereals and many corn cereals often contain wheat, as can yogurt, lunch meat and even some packages of ground beef. Even your shortening may contain vitamin E that was extracted from wheat.

Your best defense is to keep your foods lists with you when you're ordering food online or buying groceries in the supermarket.

**DID YOU KNOW?** *Another key to avoiding hidden gluten is to write to your favorite food and household product manufacturers and ask for a list of their gluten-free products; many companies have these lists available. If you write to the parent companies, such as Kraft, Johnson & Johnson and General Mills, they'll often provide you with lists for all of their subsidiaries, saving you a lot of time.*

## Gluten Is Present in Nonfood Items Too

If you're feeling overwhelmed by the vast number of food items that may contain gluten, you probably don't want to hear that it's present in a lot of inedible products too. Unfortunately, you need to be just as aware of these.

For those with celiac disease and gluten sensitivity, household items can present just as much danger as a slice of Wonder Bread. Those going gluten-free voluntarily don't need to worry about these products so much, but even very slight amounts of gluten are dangerous to people with celiac disease, gluten sensitivity or a wheat allergy.

One of the groups of household products that often contains gluten is glues and adhesives. Many brands and forms of glue and paste contain gluten, as can postage stamps, stickers and the adhesive on envelopes.

Art supplies such as paints, Play-Doh and clay often contain flour. If your child has been diagnosed with celiac disease or gluten sensitivity, be sure to check their art supplies and notify their teacher as well. You also want to check the glue, paste and stickers you have in your home. Even if your child has no problem with gluten, if you or another adult does, you'll need to take precautions. It may be best to toss what you already have and start over with products you know are gluten-free.

Cleaning agents can also contain gluten, especially dish soap, dishwasher detergent and "soft" cleansers and bar soaps. Gloves may be the answer, but latex and household gloves are often dusted with flour to make them easier to put on and remove. You can order undusted gloves from a medical supply store or find them in many drugstores. They're very inexpensive and disposable, and come in boxes of fifty or one hundred. Even if you don't usually wear gloves to wash dishes or clean the house, they're good to have if your family is not gluten-free and you'll be handling foods with gluten.

Toiletries are also a concern, especially since you have a decent chance of ingesting them by getting them on your hands and then putting your fingers on or in your mouth. These include shampoos, conditioners, lotions, facial cleansers, sun protection products, lipsticks and lip balms, and even toothpaste and mouthwash.

Again, your best defense is to call or e-mail the major manufacturers or look for a contact number on the products you already have in your house. They can usually find out for you whether the product you're using is gluten-free.

# MAKING YOUR HOME GLUTEN-FREE

There are several steps you can take to make your home gluten-free and safe for you or someone else who has celiac disease or gluten sensitivity. It's not just a matter of getting rid of products you cannot eat—although that's a huge portion of the task. Obviously, if you are going on a gluten-free diet voluntarily, without medical orders, you can be more lenient about following these guidelines.

If all of this seems like it may be unnecessarily thorough, consider this information from Alexandra Anca, MHSc, RD, who co-wrote *The Complete Gluten-Free Diet and Nutrition Guide*: "We know that one-seventieth of a slice of bread causes intestinal damage in celiac disease. The question remains, what kind of damage does ingestion of a bread-crumb cause? We don't know. If it happens daily or frequently, it will keep the inflammatory response active and the lining of the intestine will continue to be damaged. The more frequent the accidents, the less time in which your body has a chance to heal. This leads to complications and unresolved symptoms."

## Clearing Out the Kitchen

### *Get Rid of Gluten Products or Segregate Them*

If you're going to make your entire kitchen gluten-free, bundle up all your products that contain gluten, including cereals, crackers, cookies, cakes, breads and anything else that includes wheat, barley or rye in the ingredients list. You can donate unopened packages to a food bank, local church, day care center or homeless shelter. Opened packages can be passed on to friends and family who will use them. As a last resort, throw opened items away.

If you have a family, partner or roommate who will not be going gluten-free, you should at least segregate the gluten-free products from those containing gluten. If space is at a premium, you can get some storage jars or containers with tight lids in which to store your gluten-free products once they've been opened. This will protect them from cross-contamination with gluten.

### *Get a New Toaster*

If you like toast, you'll need to buy a new toaster, since it's extremely difficult to clean an already-used toaster well enough to make it safe for someone with celiac disease. This is especially important if you have others in the home who will be toasting bread containing gluten. Label yours so that everyone knows it's the designated gluten-free toaster.

If you plan to eat toast on vacation, bring your toaster with you so that you can toast your gluten-free bagels, bread and waffles. You won't be able to use the toaster that's provided in your room, vacation property or hotel's self-serve dining area.

### Buy New Jars of Condiments

Any opened condiments in your refrigerator or cabinets have most likely been contaminated with gluten crumbs, so buy a new supply of condiments, including jam and jellies, mustard, ketchup, peanut butter, margarine and mayonnaise, and anything else you enjoy using. Label your jars so that other household members know to leave them alone.

---

**DID YOU KNOW?** *Squeeze bottles of your favorite condiments are a great way to avoid cross-contamination, because you won't have spoons and knives dipping in and out of the condiments. But you'll need to tell everyone not to touch the tip of the bottle to bread containing gluten. Yes, even something as small as that can make you sick.*

---

### Replace Plastic Items and Nonstick Pans

Plastic bowls and utensils scratch easily, allowing tiny amounts of gluten to become embedded in the surface. The same is true of nonstick pots and pans. You'll need to replace these, or get a second set for gluten-free cooking. Try to get brightly colored pans that are clearly separate from what you already have, so that they're not mistakenly used to prepare foods containing gluten.

It's safe to use stainless steel or glass pans and bowls for both gluten and gluten-free foods, as long as you wash them carefully.

### Have Separate Equipment for Gluten-Free Flours

There's no way you can clean all the nooks and crannies in a flour sifter, so just buy yourself a new one and keep it in a separate spot in the kitchen. And remember, handling wheat flour in a kitchen used to prepare gluten-free food is dangerous, as wheat flour can stay airborne for hours. If you must sift wheat flour, cover or remove all gluten-free food from the area.

Unless you are able to wash it in a dishwasher, you will definitely need to buy a new colander or strainer. Those tiny holes are almost impossible to clean thoroughly by hand.

---

**DID YOU KNOW?** *Gluten-free breadcrumbs and coatings can be expensive and hard to find. Save all of the heels and unused pieces of your gluten-free bread in a tightly sealed jar or bag. Then, when you need to make meatloaf or coat a piece of fish, you'll have a safe and economical source of breadcrumbs.*

---

### Throw Away or Give Away Baking Supplies

If you have flour or baking mixes in your kitchen that contain gluten, throw them away or give them away. Handle packages of flour especially carefully to make certain you don't allow any to escape into the air—if you breathe it in and swallow a tiny bit, you'll be surprised at how sick you can get.

---

**DID YOU KNOW?** *For parents with affected kids: If other family members will still be eating snacks and treats containing gluten, store them in the cupboard above the refrigerator. It's easy for children to be tempted by these treats and hard for young ones to understand that one cookie really can hurt them.*

---

You also should get rid of any opened packages of baking supplies, such as sugar and baking soda. Although these might be fine if they're unopened, opened containers probably have some cross-contamination from your previous baking activities.

## Make Your Bathroom Safe

Many toiletries and personal care products contain hidden gluten. You'll first need to find out whether the products you have on hand are safe, and then buy any replacements you may need.

If you share your bathroom with someone who is not going gluten-free, the safest thing is for them to agree to go gluten-free when it comes to toiletries. This will prevent any accidental use of something dangerous. If that's not possible, separate your items and theirs into different medicine cabinets or vanity cupboards.

## The Rest of the House

Check your home office and craft room to make sure you've gotten rid of any glues, pastes and other adhesives that may contain gluten. Finding gluten-free envelopes is challenging, so fill a jar with water and tuck in a piece of sponge. Use this to moisten envelopes.

---

**DID YOU KNOW?** *If you're renovating your home, adding on a room or even just doing some repairs, many of the products you use may contain gluten. For example, some brands of drywall and almost all mudding or joint compounds use wheat as an ingredient. Gluten can also be included in the glue in some plywood. When you cut plywood or drywall, or a sand mudding compound, you'll be breathing (and swallowing) gluten dust, and that can lead to a reaction.*

---

Wear a full HEPA respirator (not just a dust mask) if you must do the work yourself, but you'd be better off leaving these types of home repairs to someone else. Also, even if you leave your home while the work is going on, it's best to wear gloves and a mask at home until you know the dust has been thoroughly cleaned up.

# THE BEST SUBSTITUTES FOR RYE, BARLEY AND WHEAT FLOUR

For people who can't have gluten, baked goods are often a source of disappointment instead of the enjoyable indulgence they are meant to be. The typical flours used for baking and cooking include rye, barley and wheat flours, all of which have at least a small amount of gluten. Fortunately, there are several good flour alternatives you can use to turn that cake, bread or pastry into a delicious, gluten-free dessert that even your family will enjoy. Before I get into substitutions, though, there are a couple of tips you need to know that will help your baked goods turn out better.

## Guar Gum or Xanthan Gum Help With Rise and Texture

In addition to trapping air in baked goods and making them rise well, gluten acts as a binding and emulsifying agent. In other words, it helps hold together and even disperse all the ingredients in a batter or dough. Therefore, when you remove gluten, your end product may be crumbly or grainy. A good way to help with this problem is to add one teaspoon of guar gum or xanthan gum per cup of gluten-free flour. This helps with binding and will produce a smoother texture. Measure carefully though, because if you use too much, the end product may turn out heavy or gummy.

---

**DID YOU KNOW?** *One of the secrets to successfully cooking and baking with gluten-free flour is to avoid mixing it any more than you absolutely have to, and to bake it as soon as possible. This is because gluten is a protein that traps air in the cake or bread. Gluten-free dough doesn't have that ability. If you mix gluten-free flours too much or let them sit before baking, the air will escape and your dough or batter won't rise as well as it normally should. Just use a light hand with mixing and bake immediately for maximum rise.*

---

Now let's look at some good gluten-free substitutes for your favorite flours.

## Good Flours for Baking

Because different flours interact differently with the other ingredients in a recipe, some gluten-free flours are more suited to baking than others. If you're making a cake, pizza dough or pastry, the best flours to use include rice flour, sorghum flour, tapioca flour and potato flour. Remember to add guar gum or xanthan gum so that you get a good rise and a nice texture.

It's best if you experiment and find your own preferred blends, but when you substitute flours in your favorite traditional recipes, use the following measurements per cup of wheat flour.

*Rice flour:* Substitute ¾ cup for every 1 cup wheat flour, 1 ¼ cups barley flour or 1 ⅓ cups rye flour. If you use rice flour, be aware that your baked product may have a grainy texture. Since this is one of the more readily available gluten-free flours, you may choose to accept the textural issues in favor of convenience. If possible, mix in ¼ cup of either potato or tapioca flour per cup of rice flour to improve the texture. You can also try brown rice flour, which is harder to find and a little more expensive, but also less grainy.

*Tapioca flour:* Substitute tapioca cup for cup with wheat flour. Use 1 cup tapioca for every 1 ¼ cups barley flour or 1 ⅓ cups rye flour.

*Potato flour:* Substitute ¾ cup potato flour for every 1 cup wheat flour, every 1 ¼ cups barley flour or every 1 ⅓ cups rye flour, because potato is a bit heavier. Also, if you use potato flour, remember that it has a potato-y flavor and may change the flavor of your recipe. If you're concerned about this, try mixing it with tapioca or rice flour.

*Sorghum flour:* Perhaps the best-tasting flour, this should be used in equal amounts when substituting for wheat, rye or barley flours.

## Good Substitutes for Batter

If you want to batter fish, meats or vegetables to fry or bake them, some good substitutions include corn flour or rice flour mixed with ¼ teaspoon baking powder. Don't use guar gum or xanthan gum for batters; it's not necessary.

## Good Gluten-Free Substitutions for Pancakes

Just about everybody loves pancakes, crepes and waffles for breakfast (or even for supper, for those of you who are a bit more unconventional), but people who need to go gluten-free usually have to skip them. Well, now you don't have to do that! Just substitute rice, sorghum or buckwheat flour in your pancake, crepe and waffle recipes.

Buckwheat flour is naturally gluten-free, but remember that it has a very distinctive flavor and texture. Also, make sure that when you buy it, it actually says "gluten-free," because buckwheat flour is frequently processed with the same machinery that processes wheat flour and may become contaminated. If you're making pancakes, crepes or waffles, you want them to rise, so remember to use guar gum or xanthan gum in your pancake batter, regardless of which gluten-free flour you're using.

## Choosing the Best Flour for the Job

Here are a couple basic rules to use when trying to decide which flour to use.

Medium gluten-free flours, such as brown rice flour and sorghum flour, are similar to using white, all-purpose flour.

Heavier gluten-free grain flours, such as buckwheat, millet, cornmeal and legume/bean flours, are similar to baking with whole-grain flours such as barley and rye.

> **DID YOU KNOW?** *If you can find certified gluten-free oats, you can make your own oat flour by grinding the oats in your food processor—1 ¼ cup of oats will yield about a cup of oat flour and will work as a substitute for wheat, rye or barley flour.*

When it comes right down to it, your choice of gluten-free flour substitutions is all about what tastes good to you. Experiment, try mixing the different flours and figure out what works best for your particular tastes. The fact that you can't have gluten doesn't mean you have to go without dessert or batter-fried foods. Also, several of the top prepackaged cake and dessert manufacturers now offer gluten-free options that taste great and are just as convenient to make as their gluten-containing cousins. Whatever you do though, don't think your cake and cookie days are over just because you can't have gluten.

# STRATEGIES FOR LIVING GLUTEN-FREE

L iving with a food restriction is never easy, but when you're trying to coordinate a tasty meal that everybody in the house can eat, it gets even tougher. Because so many things contain gluten, you need to be extremely careful about the ingredients you use. Fortunately, there are many options available to you that are both gluten-free and delicious. Soon you'll be making every meal a delight for the entire family without sacrificing taste or leaving anybody out.

## Plan Your Meals Ahead

This is probably the easiest thing you can do to make meal preparation easier. If you typically make spaghetti for the family on Tuesday, make gluten-free noodles to top with gluten-free spaghetti sauce instead. If your clan has requested your special fried chicken over the weekend, you can make sure you have enough roast chicken for yourself and eat the same non-gluten side dishes as the rest of the family. When you plan ahead it's easier to avoid cooking two whole separate meals.

## Keep Gluten-Free Goodies at Home

There's no reason everyone has to go without goodies just because one person has a gluten restriction. It's okay to keep cookies, cakes and breads in the house, but try to have substitutes for the person who is going gluten-free. There are many good prepackaged desserts, cookies and snacks that are both gluten-free and delicious, so keep some of these on hand so that nobody feels left out at snack time. Remember to mark all gluten-free foods with a big "GF" or other recognizable mark so that it's obvious the food is okay to eat.

## Take a Course on Gluten-Free Cooking

Expanding your repertoire of gluten-free recipes will make it easier for you to prepare gluten-free meals the whole family will love. This will save you the time and trouble of making something different for yourself.

It's also a great way to get out and meet other people and exchange ideas with those who share your challenges. By taking a course at a community college or culinary school, you'll not only learn some new techniques, but will also be able to network with other people and learn even more ways to make your life easier. Check with your local community college, because often, if there isn't an adult education course available on a given subject, they may be willing to create one if there's enough interest.

## Teach Other Family Members About the Diet

It's important that everybody in the family understands the ins and outs of a gluten-free diet. They should also know why it's so important that mom, dad, brother or sister not eat gluten, so that they will take the situation as seriously as they should. Also, be positive about it. If your child is the one with the gluten issue, they'll be learning how to deal with this restriction from you. Be sure you approach this as just another part of daily life—important, yes, but not something that should make them feel ostracized or different.

## Be Willing to Experiment

There are many tasty options out there for baking and cooking that are gluten-free. Quinoa, buckwheat flour and corn flour are all delicious as well as healthy. By experimenting with different flavors, you'll find out what works and what doesn't. As you find good recipes, be sure to save them so you can make them again. This will also make it easier for someone else to cook gluten-free for you!

## Double or Triple Up When You Cook

The hardest, most time-consuming part of cooking anything, whether it's gluten-free or not, is the preparation. If you're taking the time to cook on the weekends or on your nights off, just double up the recipes. Then all you have to do is pop the leftovers in the oven or microwave and you have an awesome, homemade meal in just a few minutes.

Gluten-free pancakes or waffles can also be made ahead of time. These are both great bread substitutes when making a sandwich and are easy for a younger child to prepare on their own. A few moments in the microwave or toaster and they have either an instant meal or a base for their sandwich.

## Strategies for Eating at Restaurants, at Parties and on Holidays

The hardest time to follow any diet may be during special occasions. By planning ahead and using these tips, you'll be able to make it through the pitfalls of a gluten-riddled environment safely, happily and with a full belly.

## Educate Yourself

As with any diet, you need to know what you can have and what you can't. Because gluten is used so widely in everything from breads to gravies and sauces, it's important that you know what foods it may be in. By educating yourself in advance, you can easily pick out menu items that are likely to be safe and then ask the server about them before you order.

## Ask for the Gluten-Free Menu

Because of the prevalence of people who can't have gluten, many restaurants now offer a gluten-free menu—so ask for it. Check out the restaurant on the Internet beforehand to see if it mentions gluten-free options. At the very least, many restaurants have their menus posted online so that you can figure out in advance what you want to order.

If all else fails, let the server know that you have can't have gluten and choose a couple of menu items for them to ask the chef about. Restaurants are generally willing to accommodate special dietary needs, so if there's a particular item that you really want, the chef may very well make you a version of it that's gluten-free. Just be sure the kitchen knows how to safely prepare gluten-free dishes without danger of cross-contamination. For instance, that means no wiping down plates with towels that have touched sauces or gravies with gluten.

## Alert Your Hosts in Advance

If your host knows in advance that you or a member of your party can't have gluten, they can make sure to include a few gluten-free foods. If you're not comfortable letting them know, make sure that you either eat before you go or take something appropriate with you.

If it's a catered party or function, you have options there, too. Many caterers specifically ask the host if there are any special dietary needs when they are discussing and planning meals. They will gladly prepare something you can have, so that you may enjoy eating with everybody else without worry. Remember, a good host wants to meet the needs of their guests and may feel bad if you don't let them know in advance so that they can be prepared.

## Teach Your Child About Eating Gluten-Free

When it comes right down to it, it's your responsibility to make sure your child knows what foods are safe to eat. Until they can learn what is and is not okay, you'll need to teach them not to eat anything without asking you first. A good alternative is to teach them what foods are acceptable to eat anytime you're out, such as vegetables and fruits, and which foods they need to either skip or ask you about. If there are snacks or appetizers placed on a buffet, take your child to the table and explain what they can have.

## Take Safe Foods With You

If you don't feel comfortable telling the host about your needs, or if you're not sure there are going to be foods available for you or your child, take something with you. This way, you know for a fact that the food is safe. This is a good idea, especially if you're going on a picnic or to an outing that's just going to have snacks.

If you're the one with the gluten allergy, you can just eat before you go, but if it's your child with the restriction, make sure you take something so that they aren't left out in case there's nothing gluten-free available. One nice thing about taking a gluten-free dish along: Other guests may be coming who also have gluten issues. Your dish might save the occasion for them, too.

## Plan Ahead

If you're throwing a party or cooking the holiday meal, plan your menu in advance, down to the last ingredient. There's nothing worse than being ready to mash the potatoes and realizing that you didn't get any gluten-free broth with which to make the gravy. A little bit of planning will make your life much easier, so take the extra time to do it right.

Living a gluten-free lifestyle isn't always easy when you're trying to do it on the go. On top of the regular stress created by just attending a party or getting the kids ready to go out, you also have to worry about whether or not there are going to be safe foods available for you or your family member. By educating yourself and planning ahead, you can take much of the stress out of the ordeal and turn it instead into the happy event that it should be.

## Substitutions to Try When the Cravings Hit

Making the transition to a gluten-free diet can be trying, especially if celiac disease or gluten sensitivity requires you to quit cold turkey and fast. Here are some substitutions you can try when you find yourself longing for a favorite meal or snack and don't have a gluten-free version on hand.

| When You Want: | Try Having: |
| --- | --- |
| Pizza | Chicken cacciatore with a layer of mozzarella |
| A chocolate malt | A chocolate protein shake or hot cocoa |
| Macaroni and cheese | A cheesy bowl of risotto |
| A roast beef sandwich from the deli | A roast beef sandwich wrapped in lettuce |
| Lemon meringue pie | Lemon yogurt or lemon pudding |
| A brownie | A square of dark chocolate |
| Hot cereal or oatmeal | Cream of Rice cereal |
| Bread pudding | Rice pudding |
| Spaghetti | Spaghetti sauce over spaghetti squash |
| Chicken noodle soup | Chicken rice or hot and sour soup |

There are a number of gluten-free versions of many of your favorite foods, and I have included some of them and where you can find them in the resources section. I've also provided recipes in the last section of this book for many safe homemade versions of American cuisine classics.

# Living a Gluten-Free Lifestyle

# (10)

## THE GOOD, THE BAD AND THE GLUTEN— WHAT YOU CAN AND CANNOT EAT

Because celiac disease and gluten sensitivity require you to avoid even the smallest amounts of hidden gluten, I've provided lists of Allowed and Not Allowed Foods and ingredients in the next chapter. The lists may be cumbersome, but they'll help you to check ingredient labels as you do your shopping.

### The Basics

To cover just the basic guidelines, you cannot have any products that contain wheat, rye, barley or anything derived from them. (If you have a wheat allergy, rye and barley may be okay for you.)

Malt is derived from barley, so you'll have to eliminate all malt products, including malted milk, Ovaltine, malt cereals, malt vinegar (including dressings and sauces that contain it) and most beer.

Unless you can find certified gluten-free oats, you cannot eat most commercial oat products, including oatmeal, oatmeal cookies, many granola and snack bars and most multigrain cereals. The problem is not necessarily with the oats themselves—some studies have shown that oats do not cause a reaction in people with celiac disease, although others studies say it depends on the person and the type of oats. More frequently, though the problem is that oats can easily be contaminated with wheat during harvest, storage or other stages of processing.

Next up are the Allowed and Not Allowed Foods Lists. It's best to print copies to keep with you. I'll give you some helpful guidelines in the shopping guide (chapter 14) to make your actual grocery shopping experience much easier.

# THE ALLOWED AND NOT ALLOWED
# FOODS LISTS

## Allowed Foods List

- Acacia gum
- Acesulfame potassium (aka Acesulfame K)
- Acetanisole
- Acetophenone
- Acorn quercus
- Adipic acid
- Adzuki bean
- Agar
- Agave
- Albumen
- Alcohol (distilled spirits, including bourbon, gin, rum, Scotch whiskey, tequila, vodka)
- Alfalfa
- Algae
- Algin
- Alginate

- Alginic acid
- Alkalized cocoa
- Allicin
- Almond nut
- Alpha-amylase
- Alpha-lactalbumin
- Aluminum
- Amaranth
- Ambergris
- Ammonium hydroxide
- Ammonium phosphate
- Ammonium sulphate
- Amylopectin
- Amylose
- Annatto
- Annatto color
- Apple cider vinegar
- Arabic gum
- Arrowroot
- Artichokes
- Artificial butter flavor
- Artificial flavoring
- Ascorbic acid
- Aspartame (may cause irritable bowel syndrome symptoms)
- Aspartic acid
- Aspic
- Astragalus gummifer
- Autolyzed yeast extract
- Avena sativia (if allowed oats)
- Avena sativia extract (if allowed oats)

- Avidin
- Azodicarbonamide
- Baking soda
- Balsamic vinegar
- Bean, adzuki
- Bean, hyacinth
- Bean, lentil
- Bean, mung
- Bean, romano (borlotti)
- Bean, tepary
- Beans
- Beeswax
- Benzoic acid
- Besan (chickpea flour)
- Beta carotene
- Beta glucan (if allowed oats)
- Betaine
- BHA
- BHT
- Bicarbonate of soda
- Biotin
- Blue cheese
- Brown sugar
- Buckwheat
- Butter (check additives)
- Butyl compounds
- Butylated hydroxyanisole
- Calcium acetate
- Calcium carbonate
- Calcium caseinate

- Calcium chloride
- Calcium disodium
- Calcium hydroxide
- Calcium lactate
- Calcium pantothenate
- Calcium phosphate
- Calcium propionate
- Calcium silicate
- Calcium sorbate
- Calcium stearate
- Calcium stearoyl lactylate
- Calcium sulfate
- Calrose
- Camphor
- Cane sugar
- Cane vinegar
- Canola (rapeseed)
- Canola oil (rapeseed oil)
- Caprylic acid
- Carageenan chondrus crispus
- Carbonated water
- Carboxymethyl cellulose
- Carmine
- Carnauba wax
- Carob bean
- Carob bean gum
- Carob flour
- Carrageenan
- Casein
- Cassava manihot esculenta

- Castor oil
- Catalase
- Cellulose[1]
- Cellulose ether
- Cellulose gum
- Cetyl alcohol
- Cetyl stearyl alcohol
- Champagne vinegar
- Chana (chickpea)
- Chana flour (chickpea flour)
- Cheeses (most, but check ingredients)
- Chestnuts
- Chickpea (garbanzo beans)
- Chlorella
- Chocolate
- Chocolate liquor
- Choline chloride
- Chromium citrate
- Chymosin
- Cider
- Citric acid
- Citrus red No. 2
- Cochineal
- Cocoa
- Cocoa butter
- Coconut
- Coconut vinegar
- Collagen
- Colloidal silicon dioxide
- Confectioners' glaze

- Copernicia cerifera
- Copper sulphate
- Corn
- Corn flour
- Corn gluten
- Corn masa flour
- Corn meal
- Corn starch
- Corn sugar
- Corn sugar vinegar
- Corn sweetener
- Corn syrup
- Corn syrup solids
- Corn vinegar
- Cortisone
- Cotton seed
- Cotton seed oil
- Cowitch
- Cowpea
- Cream of tartar
- Crospovidone
- Curds
- Cyanocobalamin
- Cysteine
- Dal (lentils)
- D-alpha-tocopherol
- Dasheen flour (taro)
- Dates
- D-calcium pantothenate
- Delactosed whey

- Demineralized whey
- Desamidocollagen
- Dextran
- Dextrose
- Diglycerides
- Dioctyl sodium
- Dioctyl sodium solfosuccinate
- Dipotassium phosphate
- Disodium guanylate
- Disodium inosinate
- Disodium phosphate
- Distilled alcohols
- Distilled vinegar
- Distilled white vinegar
- Dutch processed cocoa
- EDTA (ethylenediaminetetraacetic acid)
- Egg
- Egg yolk
- Elastin
- Ester gum
- Ethyl alcohol
- Ethyl maltol
- Ethyl vanillin
- Ethylenediaminetetraacetic acid
- Expeller pressed canola oil
- FD&C blue No. 1 dye
- FD&C blue No. 1 lake
- FD&C blue No. 2 dye
- FD&C blue No. 2 lake
- FD&C green No. 3 dye

- FD&C green No. 3 lake
- FD&C red No. 3 dye
- FD&C red No. 40 dye
- FD&C red No. 40 lake
- FD&C yellow No. 5 dye
- FD&C yellow No. 6 dye
- FD&C yellow No. 6 lake
- Ferric orthophosphate
- Ferrous fumerate
- Ferrous gluconate
- Ferrous lactate
- Ferrous sulfate
- Fish (fresh)
- Flaked rice
- Flax
- Folacin
- Folate
- Folic acid–folacin
- Formaldehyde
- Fructose
- Fruit (including dried)
- Fruit vinegar
- Fumaric acid
- Galactose
- Garbanzo beans
- Gelatin
- Glucoamylase
- Gluconolactone
- Glucose
- Glucose syrup

- Glutamate (free)
- Glutamic acid
- Glutamine (amino acid)
- Glutinous rice
- Glutinous rice flour
- Glycerides
- Glycerin
- Glycerol monooleate
- Glycol
- Glycol monosterate
- Glycolic acid
- Gram flour (chickpea)
- Grape skin extract
- Grits, corn
- Guar gum
- Gum arabic
- Gum base
- Gum tragacanth
- Gum, acacia
- Hemp
- Hemp seeds
- Herb vinegar
- Herbs
- Hexanedioic acid
- High fructose corn syrup
- Hominy
- Honey
- Hops
- Horseradish (pure)
- Hyacinth bean

- Hydrogen peroxide
- Hydrolyzed caseinate
- Hydrolyzed meat protein
- Hydrolyzed soy protein
- Hydroxypropyl cellulose
- Hydroxypropyl methylcellulose
- Hypromellose
- Illepe
- Inulin
- Invert sugar
- Iodine
- Iron ammonium citrate
- Isinglass
- Isolated soy protein
- Isomalt
- Job's tears
- Jowar (sorghum)
- Karaya gum
- Kasha (roasted buckwheat)
- K-carmine color
- Keratin
- K-gelatin
- Koshihikari (rice)
- Kudzu
- Kudzu root starch
- Lactalbumin phosphate
- Lactase
- Lactic acid
- Lactitol
- Lactose

- Lactulose
- Lanolin
- Lard
- L-cysteine
- Lecithin
- Lemon grass
- Lentils
- Licorice
- Licorice extract
- Lipase
- L-leucine
- L-lysine
- L-methionine
- Locust bean gum
- L-tryptophan
- Magnesium carbonate
- Magnesium hydroxide
- Magnesium oxide
- Maize
- Maize, waxy
- Malic acid
- Malt dextrin
- Maltol
- Manganese sulfate
- Manioc
- Masa
- Masa farina
- Masa flour
- Meat (fresh)
- Medium chain triglycerides

- Menhaden oil
- Methyl cellulose[2]
- Microcrystalline cellulose
- Micro-particulated egg white protein
- Milk
- Milk protein isolate
- Millet
- Milo (sorghum)
- Mineral oil
- Mineral salts
- Molybdenum amino acid chelate
- Mono and diglycerides
- Monocalcium phosphate
- Monoglycerides
- Monopotassium phosphate
- Monosaccharides
- Monosodium glutamate (MSG)
- Monosterate
- MSG
- Mung bean
- Musk
- Mustard flour
- Myristic acid
- Natural smoke flavor
- Neotame
- Niacin
- Niacin–niacin amide
- Nitrates
- Nitrous oxide
- Nonfat milk

- Nut, acorn
- Nut, almond
- Nuts (except wheat, rye and barley)
- Oats (only if allowed)
- Oils and fats
- Oleic acid
- Oleoresin
- Olestra
- Oleyl alcohol
- Oleyl oil
- Orange B
- Oryzanol
- Palmitic acid
- Pantothenic acid
- Papain
- Paprika
- Paraffin
- Partially hydrogenated cottonseed oil
- Partially hydrogenated soybean oil
- Pea flour
- Pea starch
- Pea, cow
- Peanut flour
- Peanuts
- Peas
- Pectin
- Pectinase
- Peppermint oil
- Peppers
- Pepsin

- Peru balsam
- Petrolatum
- PGPR (polyglycerol polyricinoleate)
- Phenylalanine
- Phosphoric acid
- Phosphoric glycol
- Pigeon peas
- Polenta
- Polydextrose
- Polyethylene glycol
- Polyglycerol
- Polyglycerol polyricinoleate (PGPR)
- Polysorbate 60
- Polysorbate 80
- Polysorbates
- Potassium benzoate
- Potassium caseinate
- Potassium citrate
- Potassium iodide
- Potassium lactate
- Potassium matabisulphite
- Potassium sorbate
- Potato flour
- Potato starch
- Potatoes
- Povidone
- Prinus
- Pristane
- Propolis
- Propyl gallate

- Propylene glycol
- Propylene glycol monosterate
- Protease
- Psyllium
- Pyridoxine hydrochloride
- Quinoa
- Ragi
- Raisin vinegar
- Rape
- Recaldent
- Reduced iron
- Rennet
- Rennet casein
- Resinous glaze
- Reticulin
- Riboflavin
- Rice
- Rice (enriched)
- Rice flour
- Rice starch
- Rice syrup
- Rice vinegar
- Ricinoleic acid
- Romano bean (borlotti)
- Rosematta rice
- Rosin
- Royal jelly
- Saccharin
- Saffron
- Sago

- Sago flour
- Sago palm
- Sago starch
- Saifun (bean threads)
- Salt
- Seaweed
- Seed, sesame
- Seed, sunflower
- Seeds (except wheat, rye and barley)
- Shea
- Sherry vinegar
- Silicon dioxide
- Soba (be sure it's 100 percent buckwheat)
- Sodium acetate
- Sodium acid pyrophosphate
- Sodium alginate
- Sodium ascorbate
- Sodium benzoate
- Sodium caseinate
- Sodium citrate
- Sodium erythrobate
- Sodium hexametaphosphate
- Sodium lactate
- Sodium lauryl sulfate
- Sodium meta-bisulphite
- Sodium nitrate
- Sodium phosphate
- Sodium polyphosphate
- Sodium silaco aluminate
- Sodium stannate

- Sodium stearoyl lactylate
- Sodium sulphite
- Sodium tripolyphosphate
- Solfosuccinate
- Sorbic acid
- Sorbitan monosterate
- Sorbitol, mannitol (may cause irritable bowl syndrome symptoms)
- Sorghum
- Sorghum flour
- Soy
- Soy lecithin
- Soy protein
- Soy protein isolate
- Soybean
- Spices (pure)
- Spirits (distilled, without malt or barley)
- Spirit vinegar
- Stearamide
- Stearamine
- Stearates
- Stearic acid
- Stearyl lactate
- Stevia
- Succotash (corn and beans)
- Sucralose
- Sucrose
- Sulfites
- Sulfur dioxide
- Sunflower seed

- Sweet chestnut flour
- Tagatose
- Tallow
- Tapioca
- Tapioca flour
- Tapioca starch
- Tara gum
- Taro
- Taro gum
- Taro root
- Tartaric acid
- Tartrazine
- TBHQ (tetra or tributylhydroquinone)
- Tea
- Tea-tree oil
- Teff
- Teff flour
- Tepary bean
- Textured vegetable protein
- Thiamine hydrochloride
- Thiamine mononitrate
- Thiamin hydrochloride
- Titanium dioxide
- Tofu (soybean curd)
- Torula yeast
- Tragacanth
- Tragacanth gum
- Triacetin
- Tri-calcium phosphate
- Trypsin

- Turmeric (kurkuma)
- TVP
- Tyrosine
- Urad/urid beans
- Urad/urid dal (peas)
- Urad/urid flour
- Vanilla extract
- Vanilla flavoring
- Vanillin
- Vinegar (all except malt)
- Vinegars (distilled)
- Vitamin A (retinol)
- Vitamin A palmitate
- Vitamin B1
- Vitamin B-12
- Vitamin B2
- Vitamin B6
- Vitamin D
- Vitamin E acetate
- Waxy maize
- Whey
- Whey protein concentrate
- Whey protein isolate
- White vinegar
- Wild rice
- Wine (and grape-based fermented beverages, such as champagne)
- Wine vinegars (distilled)
- Xanthan gum
- Xylitol

- Yam flour
- Yeast
- Yogurt (plain, unflavored)
- Zinc oxide
- Zinc sulfate

[1] The problem with caramel color is it may or may not contain gluten, depending on how it is manufactured. In the United States, caramel color must conform with FDA standards, as outlined in the Code of Federal Regulations Title 21 (21 CFR), Part 73. This regulation states: "The color additive caramel is the dark-brown liquid or solid material resulting from the carefully controlled heat treatment of the following food-grade carbohydrates: Dextrose [corn sugar], invert sugar, lactose [milk sugar], malt syrup [usually from barley malt], molasses [from sugar cane], starch hydrolysates and fractions thereof [which can include wheat], sucrose [cane or beet sugar]."

[2] If this ingredient is made in North America, it is likely to be gluten-free.

## Not Allowed Foods

- Abyssinian hard wheat (Triticum durum)
- Alcohol (non-distilled, malt beverages, rye whiskey)
- Amp-isostearoyl hydrolyzed wheat protein
- Atta flour
- Barley grass (may contain seeds)
- Barley hordeum vulgare
- Barley malt
- Beer (most contain barley or wheat)
- Bleached flour
- Bran
- Bread flour
- Brewer's yeast
- Brown flour

- Bulgur (bulgur wheat, nuts)
- Bulgur wheat
- Cereal binding
- Chilton
- Club wheat (Triticum aestivum subspecies compactum)
- Common wheat (Triticum aestivum)
- Cookie crumbs
- Cookie dough
- Cookie dough pieces
- Couscous
- Crisped rice
- Dinkle (spelt)
- Disodium oleamido peg-2 solfosuccinate
- Durum wheat (Triticum durum)
- Edible coatings
- Edible films
- Edible starch
- Einkorn (Triticum monococcum)
- Emmer (Triticum dicoccon)
- Enriched bleached flour
- Enriched bleached wheat flour
- Enriched flour
- Farina
- Farina graham
- Faro
- Filler
- Flour (normally this is wheat)
- Fu (dried wheat gluten)
- Germ
- Graham flour

- Granary flour
- Groats (barley, wheat)
- Hard wheat
- Heeng
- Hing
- Hordeum vulgare extract
- Hydrolyzed wheat gluten
- Hydrolyzed wheat protein
- Hydrolyzed wheat starch
- Hydroxypropyltrimonium hydrolyzed wheat protein
- Kamet (wheat pasta)
- Kecap manis (soy sauce)
- Ketjap manis (soy sauce)
- Kluski pasta
- Macha wheat (Triticum aestivum)
- Maida (Indian wheat flour)
- Malt
- Malt extract
- Malt flavoring
- Malt syrup
- Malt vinegar
- Malted barley flour
- Malted milk
- Matza, matzah, matzo
- Matzo meal
- Matzo semolina
- Meringue
- Meripro 711
- Mir
- Nishasta

- Oriental wheat (Triticum turanicum)
- Orzo pasta
- Pasta (made with not allowed flours)
- Pearl barley
- Persian wheat (Triticum carthlicum)
- Perungayam
- Polish wheat (Triticum polonicum)
- Poulard wheat (Triticum turgidum)
- Rice malt (if barley or koji are used)
- Roux
- Rusk
- Rye
- Seitan
- Semolina
- Semolina triticum
- Shot wheat (Triticum aestivum)
- Small spelt
- Spelt (Triticum spelta)
- Spirits (non-distilled)
- Sprouted wheat or barley
- Stearyldimonium hydroxypropyl hydrolyzed wheat protein
- Strong flour
- Suet in packets
- Tabbouleh
- Tabouli
- Teriyaki sauce
- Timopheevii wheat (Triticum timopheevii)
- Triticale x triticosecale
- Triticum vulgare (wheat) flour lipids
- Triticum vulgare (wheat) germ extract

- Triticum vulgare (wheat) germ oil
- Udon (wheat noodles)
- Unbleached flour
- Vavilovi wheat (Triticum aestivum)
- Vital wheat gluten
- Wheat (Triticum vulgare) bran extract
- Wheat amino acids
- Wheat bran extract
- Wheat germ extract
- Wheat germ glycerides
- Wheat germ oil
- Wheat germ, amidopropyldimonium hydroxypropyl hydrolyzed wheat protein
- Wheat grass (may contain seeds)
- Wheat nuts
- Wheat protein
- Wheat, Abyssinian hard (Triticum durum)
- Wheat, bulgur
- Wheat (Durum triticum)
- Wheat (Triticum aestivum)
- Wheat (Triticum monococcum)
- Whole-meal flour
- Wild einkorn (Triticum boeotictim)
- Wild emmer (Triticum dicoccoides)

## Foods That Require Caution

The following items may or may not contain gluten, depending on where and how they are made. It is sometimes necessary to check with the manufacturer to find out.

Artificial color[3]
Baking powder[3]
Caramel color[1,2]
Caramel flavoring[1,2]
Clarifying agents[3]
Coloring[3]
Dextrimaltose[1,6]
Dextrins[1,6]
Dry-roasted nuts[3]
Emulsifiers[3]
Enzymes[3]
Fat replacer[3]
Flavoring[5]
Food starch modified[1,3]
Food starch[1,3]
Glucose syrup[3]
Gravy cubes[3]
Ground spices[3]
HPP[4]
HVP[4]
Hydrogenated starch hydrolysate[3]
Hydrolyzed plant protein[3]
Hydrolyzed protein[3]
Hydrolyzed vegetable protein[3]
Hydroxy-propylated starch[3]
Maltose[3]
Miso[3]
Mixed tocopherols[3]
Modified food starch[1,3]
Modified starch[1,3]
Natural flavoring[5]

Natural flavors[5]
Natural juices[3]
Non-dairy creamer[3]
Pre-gelatinized starch[3]
Protein hydrolysates[3]
Seafood analogs[3]
Seasonings[3]
Sirimi[3]
Smoke flavoring[3]
Soba noodles[3]
Soy sauce solids[3]
Soy sauce[3]
Sphingolipids[3]
Stabilizers[3]
Starch[1,3]
Stock cubes[3]
Suet[4]
Tocopherols[3]
Vegetable broth[3]
Vegetable gum[3]
Vegetable protein[3]
Vegetable starch[3]
Vitamins[3]
Wheat starch[4]

[1] If this ingredient is made in North America, it is likely to be gluten-free.

[2] The problem with caramel color is it may or may not contain gluten, depending on how it is manufactured. In the United States, caramel color must conform with FDA standards, as outlined in the Code of Federal Regulations Title 21 (21 CFR), Part 73. This regulation states: "The color additive caramel is the dark-brown liquid or solid material resulting from the carefully controlled heat treatment of the following food-grade carbohydrates: Dextrose [corn sugar], invert sugar, lactose [milk sugar], malt syrup [usually from barley malt], molasses [from sugar

cane], starch hydrolysates and fractions thereof [which can include wheat], sucrose [cane or beet sugar]."

[3] May use a grain or byproduct containing gluten in the manufacturing process, or as an ingredient.

[4] Most celiac disease support organizations in the United States and Canada do not believe that wheat starch is safe for people with celiac disease. In Europe, however, most doctors and celiac disease support organizations consider Codex Alimentarius Quality wheat starch acceptable in the celiac diet. This is a higher quality of wheat starch than is generally available in the United States or Canada.

[5] According to 21 CFR, Section 101.22: "The term natural flavor or natural flavoring means the essential oil, oleoresin, essence or extractive, protein hydrolysate, distillate, or any product of roasting, heating or enzymolysis, which contains the flavoring constituents derived from a spice, fruit or fruit juice, vegetable or vegetable juice, edible yeast, herb, bark, bud, root, leaf or similar plant material, meat, seafood, poultry, eggs, dairy products, or fermentation products thereof, whose significant function in food is flavoring rather than nutritional."

[6] Dextrin is an incompletely hydrolyzed starch. It is prepared by dry-heating corn, waxy maize, waxy milo, potato, arrowroot, wheat, rice, tapioca, or sago starches, or by dry-heating the starches after treatment with safe and suitable alkalis, acids, or pH control agents, and drying the acid- or alkali-treated starch. Therefore, unless you know the source, you must avoid dextrin.

$$\left(12\right)$$

## THE GLUTEN-FREE SHOPPING GUIDE

Grocery shopping can be a real chore when you're on a gluten-free diet, especially when you're first starting out. There can be a lot of new things to learn and to buy. Be prepared to take more time shopping, and also try to remember that in a short time you will learn which brands and products are safe to buy and be able to shop almost as quickly, if not just as quickly, as you did before.

Follow these guidelines and hints to help you cover your bases and streamline your grocery shopping. Doing so will help make the process less stressful.

### Make a Shopping Notebook

This is one of the very best steps you can take, and your notebook will become an invaluable tool. A notebook that has some pockets is best. An old agenda or Day Runner–type book is great, and one that fits in your handbag will be most convenient.

Print out this shopping guide and your Allowed and Not Allowed Foods Lists, reduce them if necessary, and punch holes on the paper so you can put them into your notebook.

You'll also want pages for your menu planning and grocery lists.

Add printed copies of gluten-free product lists you've obtained from food companies or celiac websites, and also a couple of blank pieces of paper to add products and brands you find in the store.

**DID YOU KNOW?** *When you call the food companies for gluten-free product lists, don't forget to ask if they have any coupons for gluten-free items. Many companies offer coupons but don't include them in the newspaper inserts. Most will put you on a monthly mailing list for coupons, which can save you a great deal of money.*

## Decide Where You're Going to Do Your Shopping

Most supermarkets have a gluten-free section in addition to the gluten-free products spread throughout the store. Some grocery stores, particularly health food stores, tend to have a wider selection. If running to more than one store is a hassle, consider ordering your gluten-free products from one of the online retailers in the resource guide and going to the supermarket only for fresh foods or foods that don't normally contain gluten anyway.

Check your supermarket's website to see if they have a list of gluten-free products they stock. Many stores offer these lists online as a service to their customers. If they don't have one on their website, ask the manager next time you shop. If your store has a list of gluten-free products, keep it in your notebook.

## Make a Menu for the Week

Try to make a menu consisting mostly of recipes that use whole, fresh foods like meats, fresh seafood and fresh produce. This will allow for more flexibility in your menu planning. You'll also save money by not having to purchase a long list of gluten-free specialty products.

## Make a Grocery List

Use the weekly menu as your guide. See what ingredients you need to purchase to make those meals and add them to your list.

Now, organize your shopping list. Some people like alphabetical lists, while others prefer to sort their lists by category and still others arrange their lists by grocery store aisle. Do what works for you, but definitely take the time to make a list. You can even create a master list and print several copies to save rewriting everything each week.

Keep your grocery list in your notebook. Having the list on hand will save you time and aggravation.

## Keep It Fresh to Keep It Fast

Fresh meats, seafood and produce should be your staples. They don't require reading the labels (except possibly for ground beef) and they're better for you. The more you buy of these ingredients, the less time and money you'll have to spend in the packaged food sections.

## Beat the Crowds

Try to pick a day and time to go shopping that is not as crowded. This will help balance out the extra time you'll spend reading labels. And if you have a question about gluten-free options, you may be more likely to find someone in the store who can help.

## Make It Easy for Yourself

Shopping every one or two weeks is usually more economical and convenient, but is only possible if you plan ahead. If you are not the type to plan ahead, you may have to shop more frequently.

# (13)

# THE GLUTEN-FREE RESOURCE GUIDE

There is a wide variety of informational websites, online retailers and recipe sites that can help make your transition to a gluten-free diet a lot easier. Here are just a few places to look for the latest information, gluten-free products, gluten-free recipes and more. In time, you'll find quite a few of your own favorites to add to the list.

## Websites for Information About Celiac Disease, Gluten Sensitivity and Gluten-Free Living

### Celiac.com
*www.celiac.com*

This is a huge informational site that has a number of articles you can download that can help you transition to a gluten-free diet. They also keep track of and post relevant news, such as product ingredient changes and labeling regulation news. This is an excellent resource for recipes as well, and you can get to The Gluten-Free Mall from the home page. Their extensive foods lists helped me put together the Allowed and Not Allowed Foods Lists in this book.

### Celiac Disease Foundation
*www.celiac.org*

A great nonprofit organization providing information, resources and news about celiac disease and gluten sensitivity.

### National Foundation for Celiac Awareness
*www.celiaccentral.org*

Another nonprofit site that has a wealth of information for both celiac disease and gluten sensitivity. A good site for news and new research findings.

## Online Food Companies and Gluten-Free Supermarkets

### The Gluten-Free Mall
*www.celiac.com/glutenfreemall/*

A very well respected gluten-free online supermarket, The Gluten-free Mall offers a wide selection of gluten-free, wheat-free, casein-free and other allergy-related health foods and special dietary products. This is an excellent resource for toiletries and vitamins, too.

### Abe's Market
*www.abesmarket.com*

Abe's Market offers a very large selection of gluten-free products and baked goods, and also offers free shipping on every order.

### Gluten Free Palace
*www.glutenfreepalace.com*

This is a gluten-free supermarket with a huge variety of gluten-free groceries available, including bagels, muffins and pasta.

## GlutenFree.com

*www.glutenfree.com*

Another gluten-free supermarket offering a very good selection. This site is very well regarded in the gluten-free online community.

## Dietary Specialties

*www.dietspec.com*

Dietary Specialties offers prepared foods such as gluten-free chicken nuggets, fish sticks, ravioli and pierogies. It's a good option for those with limited time to cook or kids with celiac disease, as it sells quite a few kid-friendly items.

## Pure Foods Gluten Free

*www.glutenfreemeals.com*

Gluten-free meals pre-cooked and delivered fresh (not frozen) by FedEx.

## Katz Gluten Free

*www.katzglutenfree.com*

A kosher gluten-free bakery providing breads, cakes, pies, pastries and rugalach.

## Everybody Eats Katz Gluten Free

*www.everybodyeats-inc.com*

Everybody Eats is a New York City restaurant that specializes in a gluten-free, nut-free menu. It delivers in New York and also ships nationwide via FedEx. It offers a number of entrees, including breads, pastas, desserts and sweets.

## Grandma Ferdon's

*www.grandmaferdons.com*

Grandma Ferdon's is a food manufacturing company with several locations in the Midwestern United States that offers 100% guaranteed gluten-free foods, including pizza, frozen dough, flours, pastries, mixes, and spices. It also offers a variety of "comfort meals" through its website.

## Kinnikinnick Foods

*www.kinnikinnick.com*

Kinnikinnick Foods makes gluten-free and casein-free foods in its own dedicated gluten-free facility, and offers a very good selection of gluten-free products. Its main line focuses on bread products, muffins, buns and rolls, breakfast items (including frozen waffles) and donuts.

## Free From Market

*www.freefrommarket.com*

Free From Market is a specialty food store that carries close to 3,000 gluten-free items. It's a good resource for household cleaners and toiletries as well.

## Safely Gluten Free

*www.safelyglutenfree.com*

Safely Gluten Free has a wide variety of flours, pastas, pastries, cereals and more that you can order from the website. This is a great source for baking needs.

## Gluten Solutions

*www.glutensolutions.com*

Offers an array of gluten-free products, including toiletries and household items, as well as food.

## Gluten-Free Recipe Resources

These sites offer thousands of recipes for gluten-free meals and snacks.

### Allrecipes.com
*www.allrecipes.com*

This clearinghouse of user-submitted recipes has a huge selection of gluten-free recipes from which to choose.

### Tastes of Home
*www.tasteofhome.com*

This site, like the magazine it complements, has a gigantic selection of recipes, all of which include photographs. You can save your favorites to your own online recipe box or even print out 3 x 5 recipe cards. This site has an excellent selection of gluten-free meals.

### Living Without
*www.livingwithout.com*

Living Without is one of the few print magazines that centers on gluten-free living. You can subscribe to the magazine or just access a very nice selection of articles and recipes online. One great bonus is that it features lactose-free recipes as well.

### Food.com
*www.food.com*

This huge mainstream site has a pretty good selection of gluten-free recipes. You can register to make use of the "Favorites" feature, which is handy for meal planning.

## Gluten-Free Communities and Forums

Connecting with others who are on a gluten-free diet can go a long way toward easing frustration and lessening confusion. Make friends and get your questions answered by those who have been on a gluten-free diet for some time. I highly recommend taking part in some form of community or group, either online or off, as you make the transition to a gluten-free lifestyle.

Both Celiac.com and GlutenFree.com offer member forums. You can also try:

- Gluten-Free Faces, *www.glutenfreefaces.com*
- Gluten Free and Beyond, *www.glutenfreeandbeyond.org*

## (14)

# SAMPLE MEAL PLANS FOR A
# GLUTEN-FREE DIET

The best meal plan for you will depend on several things, such as the time you have to spend cooking and whether you need to lose weight while on the gluten-free diet.

I've provided different meal plans to use as a starting point to create your own menus and divided them into:

- A meal plan for the gluten-free cook
- A meal plan for people with busy schedules
- A meal plan for losing weight on a gluten-free diet

Although I've provided some recipes for gluten-free meals, desserts and snacks in Section Four, these are not intended to be staples of your daily diet. Most people already know how to make their favorite traditionally gluten-free meals, such as steak and mashed potatoes, but are concerned that they'll never be able to enjoy things like pasta, pizza, or brownies again. The recipes in the cookbook are intended to help you keep enjoying those foods that traditionally contain gluten.

Note: Dishes marked with [*] are recipes included in The Gluten-Free Diet Cookbook in Section 4.

# A Meal Plan for the Gluten-Free Cook

## Breakfast
- 1 Morning Burrito*
- 1 sliced mango
- Coffee or tea

## Morning Snack
- 1 stick mozzarella string cheese
- 1 fresh orange

## Lunch
- Tuna Stuffed Avocado*
- Tea or juice

## Afternoon Snack
- 1 fresh apple

## Dinner
- Meat Loaf*
- Roasted asparagus with lemon pepper
- 1 cup brown rice

## Dessert
- 1 Brownie*

# A Meal Plan for People With Busy Schedules

## Breakfast
- ½ cup gluten-free oats with blueberries and almond milk
- Coffee or tea
- 1 banana

## Morning Snack
- 1 fresh apple
- 1 stick mozzarella string cheese

## Lunch
- Turkey, tomato, spinach and gluten-free mayonnaise in a lettuce wrap
- 1 fresh orange
- Juice or water

## Afternoon Snack
- 6 gluten-free crackers
- 3 slices cheddar cheese

## Dinner
- Quick Fish Florentine*
- 1 cup roasted carrots
- Spinach salad with vinaigrette
- 1 gluten-free dinner roll
- Juice or tea

## Dessert
- 2 Chocolate Chip Cookies*

# A Meal Plan for Losing Weight on a Gluten-Free Diet

## Breakfast
- ½ cup gluten-free oats with almond milk
- ½ cup sliced fresh strawberries
- 1 hardboiled egg
- Coffee or tea

## Morning Snack
- 1 slice turkey breast rolled in 1 slice mozzarella
- 1 fresh peach

## Lunch
- Grilled chicken salad, made with 1 cup diced chicken breast, 1 cup fresh spinach, sliced tomato, sliced mushrooms
- 2 tablespoons light vinaigrette dressing
- Water or tea

## Afternoon Snack
- 1 sliced apple
- 1 tablespoon almond butter for dipping

## Dinner
- 1 cup Lentil Garden Soup*
- Salad made with romaine lettuce, sliced red onion, diced red pepper
- 2 tablespoons light vinaigrette

## Dessert
- ½ cup gluten-free sorbet or sherbet

# The Gluten-Free Diet Cookbook

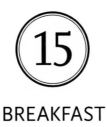

# BREAKFAST

## Fruit-Filled Crepes

*Berries are as delicious as they are healthy. A tiny bit of rice flour is used to thicken the juices of the fruit. If desired, top with a dollop of yogurt or whipped cream.*

- 2 cups frozen mixed berries
- 1 tablespoon honey
- 1 teaspoon rice flour
- Dash of cinnamon
- 1 recipe Versatile Crepes

Combine fruit, honey, flour and cinnamon in a large skillet and simmer gently over low heat for 4 minutes until thickened.

Lay the crepes out on a work surface. Spoon filling down the middle of each crepe and fold in half, then transfer to a plate.

*Serves 4*

## Versatile Crepes

*These basic crepes can be used with savory or sweet fillings. Sorghum flour and potato starch are good substitutes for all-purpose wheat flour in this recipe. Store crepes in the refrigerator for three days, or in the freezer for up to a month.*

- ½ cup sorghum flour
- ½ cup potato starch (also known as potato starch flour)
- Pinch of salt
- ½ teaspoon sugar

- 2 eggs
- ½ cup milk
- ½ cup water
- 2 tablespoons canola oil plus 2 teaspoons, divided

Use a whisk to combine flour, starch, salt and sugar in a large bowl.

In another bowl, whisk eggs, milk, water and 2 tablespoons oil. Stir into flour until well mixed.

In a 9-inch skillet, heat ½ teaspoon oil over medium heat and brush to cover the whole pan. Pour in ¼ cup of batter for each crepe, turning the pan so that the batter evenly covers the entire bottom of the pan.

Cook until the edges start to curl up, about 1 minute. Flip the crepe over and cook for another minute or until golden. Set aside on a plate to keep warm. Cook the rest of the batter, adjusting the heat and adding ½ teaspoon of oil as needed between crepes.

*Makes 10 crepes*

## Morning Burritos

*This recipe is a twist on the classic breakfast burrito. These burritos are made with crepes rather than flour tortillas. Eat them with a knife and fork—they are too delicate to pick up.*

- 1 teaspoon canola oil
- 4 eggs, beaten
- 2 tablespoons green chilies, chopped
- 1 cup grated cheddar cheese, divided
- 1 cup canned black beans, rinsed and drained
- ½ cup salsa
- 8 Versatile Crepes

Heat oil in nonstick skillet and add the eggs. Stir in chilies and cook until the eggs are almost set. Add ½ cup cheese and transfer eggs to a plate to keep warm.

Put beans and salsa into skillet, mashing the beans as they heat through.

Lay the crepes out on a work surface. Fill each crepe with eggs, beans and remaining cheese. Top with salsa and roll up to serve.

*Serves 4*

## Cheese Blintzes

*Another great breakfast entrée, cheese blintzes are rich and satisfying. Crepes are the traditional wrapper for blintzes. Use low-fat or light cream cheese if you are watching calories.*

- Nonstick cooking spray
- 1 cup ricotta cheese
- 1 (3-ounce) package cream cheese, softened
- ¼ cup sugar
- 1 teaspoon lemon juice
- 1 teaspoon lemon zest
- 1 recipe Versatile Crepes
- 1 ½ cups fresh sliced fruit or berries

Preheat oven to 350 degrees. Spray a 9 x 12-inch baking dish with nonstick cooking spray.

Mix together cheeses, sugar, juice and zest in a large bowl.

Lay the crepes out on a work surface. Spoon about 1 tablespoon cheese mixture into the center of a crepe. Fold the bottom quarter of the crepe up and over the filling. Then fold the two sides of the crepe over the filling and the bottom fold. Finally, fold the top quarter of the crepe down to form a packet. Place seam side down in the baking dish. Repeat with all the crepes.

Transfer baking dish to the oven and heat for 15 minutes. Serve topped with fruit.

*Serves 4*

## Quick-Rising Bread

*This style of quick bread needs no time to rise because it has no yeast. Potato starch and rice flour are used in place of wheat flour. Use this bread for toasting or making French toast.*

- Nonstick cooking spray
- 6 eggs, separated, at room temperature
- 3 tablespoons sugar
- ½ cup rice flour
- ¼ cup potato starch flour
- 2 teaspoons baking powder
- 1 teaspoon salt

Preheat oven to 350 degrees. Spray a 8 x 4-inch loaf pan with nonstick cooking spray.

In a large bowl, beat the egg whites until they begin to form mounds. Beat in the sugar, 1 tablespoon at a time.

In a separate bowl, beat the egg yolks at high speed for about 5 minutes until light and fluffy.

Sift together the flours, baking powder and salt. Sprinkle about one-third of the flour mixture over the egg whites and fold in gently. Repeat until all flour is incorporated. Carefully fold in the egg yolks until well blended.

Pour the batter into prepared loaf pan and bake for 45 to 50 minutes. Cool on rack in pan for 1 hour. Remove from pan and allow bread to cool for 3 more hours before slicing.

*Makes 1 loaf*

## French Toast

*French toast is a great breakfast dish to serve on weekends or for company. Gluten-free bread can become stale quickly, and this is a good way to use it up. Serve dusted with powdered sugar or drizzled with syrup.*

- 1 egg
- ½ cup milk
- ½ teaspoon pure vanilla extract
- ½ teaspoon cinnamon
- 4 teaspoons butter or margarine, divided
- 4 slices stale Quick-Rising Bread, cut in half

Beat egg, milk, vanilla and cinnamon in shallow bowl until frothy.

Heat a nonstick skillet and add 1 teaspoon butter.

Dip 2 half slices of bread into the egg mixture. Add bread to skillet and cook, turning once when the bottoms begin to brown. When both sides are browned, transfer to a plate.

Repeat dipping and cooking the French toast, melting another teaspoon of butter between batches until all slices are cooked.

*Serves 4*

# Granola

*Crunchy granola is a fruity and nutty treat. A nutrient- and calorie-rich food, it is best enjoyed in small doses. Use as a topping for yogurt, as an ingredient in granola bars or for crumb pie crusts.*

- Nonstick cooking spray
- 5 cups puffed rice cereal
- 1 cup old-fashioned rolled oats, certified gluten-free
- 1 cup raisins
- ½ cup slivered almonds
- ½ cup unsweetened, shredded coconut
- ½ cup raw sunflower seeds
- ¼ cup sesame seeds
- 1 teaspoon cinnamon
- ½ teaspoon salt
- ½ cup honey
- ¼ cup canola oil

Preheat oven to 300 degrees. Spray a large roasting pan with nonstick cooking spray.

Mix all dry ingredients together in a large bowl until well combined.

Heat the honey and oil in a small saucepan until hot but not boiling. Drizzle the honey and oil mixture over the dry ingredients and stir well with a wooden spoon to coat evenly.

Transfer mixture to the pan. Bake for 30 minutes. Turn off the oven and let the granola cool for several hours or overnight. Crumble and store in zip top bags. Store for up to 1 week.

*Makes 8–10 cups*

## Granola Bars

*Granola bars are perfect for on-the-go snacking. These rich and chewy bars use a gluten-free granola as their base. Enjoy granola bars with milk or fresh fruit.*

- Nonstick cooking spray
- ¾ cup brown sugar
- ½ cup sweetened condensed milk
- 2 tablespoons melted butter
- 1 teaspoon pure vanilla extract
- 4 cups Granola, chopped to coarse crumbs in food processor

Preheat oven to 350 degrees. Spray a 9 x 13-inch pan with nonstick cooking spray.

Mix brown sugar, condensed milk, butter and vanilla together in a bowl. Pour over the granola crumbs and mix well.

Oil your hands and press the mixture into the prepared pan. Bake for 20 minutes. Let cool for 10 minutes, then cut into 1 ½ x 3-inch bars. Store in snack-size plastic bags.

*Makes 36 bars*

# Banana Nut Bread

*Tender banana nut bread is a family favorite. A combination of soy flour, potato starch and rice flour are used in place of wheat flour. Allow this bread to cool completely before slicing. Spread with cream cheese or butter, if desired.*

- 1 cup soy flour
- ½ cup potato starch (also known as potato starch flour)
- ½ cup rice flour
- 1 ¼ teaspoons cream of tartar
- ½ teaspoon salt
- ¼ teaspoon baking soda

- ½ cup butter or margarine, softened
- ¾ cup light brown sugar
- 2 eggs, beaten until light
- ½ cup ripe bananas, mashed
- ½ cup walnuts, chopped

Preheat oven to 350 degrees. Grease an 8 x 4-inch loaf pan.

Sift together the flours, cream of tartar, salt and baking soda in a medium mixing bowl and set aside.

With an electric mixer, cream the butter in a large mixing bowl. Gradually add the sugar, beating until fluffy. Add the eggs and beat well.

Add ½ cup of the sifted flours, beating well until smooth. Add a portion of the mashed bananas, and beat until smooth. Continue alternating dry ingredients and bananas until all ingredients are fully incorporated. Stir in the nuts.

Pour into the prepared loaf pan, transfer to the oven and bake for 1 hour. Let cool on a rack before slicing and serving.

*Makes 1 loaf*

## Poppy Seed Muffins

*Lemon and poppy seeds are a classic combination. Rice flour is a basic gluten-free flour that works well in muffins. Serve these muffins hot, fresh out of the oven.*

- ¼ cup sugar
- 2 tablespoons butter, softened
- 2 eggs
- 1 cup rice flour
- 2 teaspoons baking powder
- ¼ teaspoon salt
- ½ cup milk
- 1 tablespoon poppy seeds
- ½ teaspoon lemon extract

Preheat oven to 350 degrees. Grease a muffin tin or use paper liners.

Cream sugar and butter together in a large mixing bowl with a wooden spoon. Beat in the eggs, one at a time, until thoroughly combined.

In a separate bowl, sift together the flour, baking powder and salt.

Add a portion of the sifted ingredients to the egg mixture, mixing well to combine. Add a portion of the milk and mix well. Continue alternating between sifted ingredients and milk until all ingredients are well incorporated.

Stir in the poppy seeds and lemon extract.

Portion out batter into the muffin tin or paper liners. Transfer to the oven and bake for 20 minutes, or until a toothpick inserted into a muffin comes out clean.

*Makes 12 muffins*

## Cheese Grits

*Cheesy grits are a Southern breakfast treat. Make sure your grits are gluten-free. Serve with eggs or sausage.*

- 4 cups milk
- 1 cup gluten-free grits
- ¼ cup butter
- 2 cups Monterey Jack cheese, grated
- 1 egg, beaten lightly
- 1 teaspoon salt
- ¼ teaspoon cayenne pepper
- ¼ cup Parmesan cheese, grated

Preheat oven to 350 degrees. Lightly oil an 11 x 7-inch baking dish.

In a saucepan over medium heat, bring milk just to a boil. Whisk in grits and butter gradually and smoothly. Reduce heat and simmer, stirring constantly, until grits are cooked. Remove from heat and stir in Monterey Jack cheese, egg, salt and pepper.

Pour into baking dish and sprinkle evenly with Parmesan cheese. Cover the baking dish with foil and bake for 35 minutes, or until set.

*Serves 4*

## Breakfast Hash

*Hash is a combination of meat and vegetables fried in a skillet, and is a great way to use leftovers. This recipe uses apple instead of the traditional potato. Serve with gluten-free gravy or ketchup, if desired.*

- 2 teaspoons canola oil
- ¼ cup onion, chopped
- 1 cup cooked turkey or chicken, chopped
- 1 tart apple, cored and chopped
- ½ teaspoon dried sage
- Salt and pepper to taste
- 2 eggs
- 1 tablespoon fresh parsley, chopped

Heat a large nonstick skillet and add oil. Add onion and cook until translucent.

In a large bowl, mix the meat, apple, sage, salt and pepper. Add to onion and stir well. Cook until meat is heated through and apple has softened.

Make 2 wells in the hash with the back of a spoon and carefully crack in the eggs. Cover and cook until whites are firm and yolks have cooked to desired consistency. Garnish with parsley.

*Serves 2*

## Winter Fruit Compote

*A winter fruit compote uses reconstituted dried fruit. Fruit helps supply fiber that is usually found in grains in conventional diets. Serve compote hot over cereal or pancakes.*

- ½ cup pitted prunes
- ½ cup dried apples
- ½ cup dried cherries
- ½ teaspoon cinnamon
- ¼ teaspoon powdered ginger
- Pinch of salt

Place the fruit, spices and salt in a saucepan and cover with water. Bring to a boil over medium heat. Reduce heat and simmer for 5 minutes.

Turn off the heat and allow the fruit to absorb the liquid for 2 hours, or until fruit is plump.

*Serves 4*

## Quick Skillet Scramble

*This skillet scramble is easier than an omelet but just as delicious. Make sure your bacon is gluten-free. Serve with gluten-free biscuits or toast.*

- 3 strips gluten-free bacon, diced
- 3 eggs, beaten

- Salt and pepper to taste
- ¼ cup Monterey Jack cheese, diced

In a large nonstick skillet, cook bacon over medium-low heat until crisp. Drain bacon on paper towels. Pour off most of the bacon drippings and add eggs to the pan. Season with salt and pepper.

Cook over low heat, stirring until eggs are almost set, then sprinkle on the cheese and allow to melt.

Transfer eggs to plates and garnish with bacon.

*Serves 2*

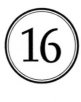

# LUNCH

## Manhattan Clam Chowder

*Manhattan clam chowder is red with tomatoes and lighter than Boston-style chowder. There is no flour to thicken Manhattan clam chowder, or other ingredients with hidden gluten. Serve with a green salad or gluten-free crackers.*

- 2 cups vegetable broth
- 1 (28-ounce) can diced tomatoes, undrained
- 2 (6 ½-ounce) cans minced clams, undrained
- 1 cup potatoes, peeled and cubed
- 1 cup onion, chopped
- ⅔ cup celery, chopped
- ½ cup green pepper, chopped
- 1 tablespoon extra virgin olive oil
- ½ teaspoon salt
- ½ teaspoon thyme
- ¼ teaspoon pepper, or to taste

Place all ingredients in slow cooker, cover and set timer to cook on low for 6 hours.

*Serves 4*

## Lentil Garden Soup

*Nourishing lentil soup is thick and satisfying. Beans and legumes are a good source of fiber and are naturally gluten-free. Serve this soup with a salad and gluten-free bread.*

- 6 cups vegetable broth
- 1 cup dried lentils, washed
- 1 tablespoon extra virgin olive oil
- 2 cups onion, chopped
- 2 cloves garlic, minced
- 2 cups fresh or canned tomatoes, chopped
- 1 cup carrots, sliced
- 1 bay leaf
- 1 teaspoon dried thyme
- ½ teaspoon dried marjoram
- Salt and pepper, to taste

In a large soup pot, bring broth and lentils to a boil over high heat. Reduce heat, cover and simmer for 30 minutes.

Meanwhile, heat a small skillet and add the olive oil. Add the onions and garlic and cook over medium heat. When they become golden, add to lentils.

Add remaining ingredients to the soup pot and cook for another 30 minutes, or until lentils and vegetables are tender. Season to taste with salt and pepper.

*Serves 4*

# Crunchy Chicken Salad

*This Asian-inspired salad is hearty with chicken and healthy vegetables. Use gluten-free tamari sauce if you cannot find gluten-free soy sauce. Serve this salad for lunch or dinner.*

- 2 cups baby salad greens, washed
- 1 cup broccoli florets, blanched and rinsed in cold water
- 1 cup cauliflower florets, blanched and rinsed in cold water
- ½ cup fresh snow peas, trimmed
- ½ red onion, sliced thin
- ¼ cup gluten-free soy sauce
- 1 tablespoon cider vinegar
- 1 tablespoon extra virgin olive oil
- 1 teaspoon honey
- 1 teaspoon sesame seeds, toasted
- 1 cup cooked chicken, cubed

Toss greens, broccoli, cauliflower, snow peas and onions in large bowl.

Whisk soy sauce, vinegar, olive oil, honey and sesame seeds in a small bowl and pour over greens. Toss salad and transfer to plates. Top each portion with chicken.

*Serves 4*

# Spinach Quiche

*A traditional quiche is a French custard baked in a crust. This lighter version of quiche has no crust and no heavy cream. Serve it with a sliced tomato salad.*

- 1 tablespoon extra-virgin olive oil
- 1 onion, chopped
- 1 (10-ounce) package frozen chopped spinach, thawed and drained
- 3 cups Monterey Jack or fontina cheese, shredded
- 5 eggs, beaten
- ½ cup milk
- ¼ teaspoon salt
- ¼ teaspoon pepper
- ¼ teaspoon nutmeg

Preheat oven to 350 degrees. Lightly oil a 9-inch pie pan.

Heat the olive oil in a large skillet over medium heat and cook the onions until soft. Squeeze spinach until very dry, then add to the onions and cook until just warmed through.

In a large bowl, combine the cheese, eggs, milk, salt, pepper and nutmeg. Add spinach and onions and mix well.

Pour the mixture into the pie pan and transfer to the oven. Bake for 30 minutes, until the eggs have set. Cool before serving.

*Serves 4*

## Tuna Stuffed Avocado

*This vibrant version of tuna salad has no mayonnaise. Add chopped green onions or capers for variety. Serve with gluten-free French bread.*

- 1 avocado, halved and pitted
- 2 teaspoons fresh lemon juice
- 1 can water-packed tuna, drained
- 1 stalk celery, thinly sliced
- 2 tablespoons fresh cilantro or parsley, chopped
- 1 teaspoon extra virgin olive oil
- Pinch cayenne pepper

Scoop the avocado flesh into a large bowl and chop roughly; reserve the shells.

Sprinkle flesh with lemon juice. Flake the tuna into the avocado and toss. Add celery, cilantro, olive oil and cayenne, and toss to combine.

Fill the avocado shells with the tuna mixture and serve.

*Serves 2*

# Springtime Chicken Soup

*Spring asparagus, peas, spinach and chives add freshness to this chicken soup. Cornstarch is a good thickener and is gluten-free. Serve this soup with a green salad and gluten-free French bread.*

- 1 (32-ounce) carton chicken broth
- 1 (10-ounce) package frozen peas and pearl onions
- 1 carrot, peeled and sliced thin
- 1 bunch asparagus, trimmed and cut into 1-inch pieces
- 1 cup fresh spinach, chopped
- ½ teaspoon dried marjoram
- ½ teaspoon salt
- ¼ teaspoon pepper
- ¼ teaspoon ground nutmeg
- 1 cup cooked chicken, diced
- ¼ cup cold water
- 2 tablespoons cornstarch
- ½ cup chives, chopped

Bring broth to a boil in a soup pot over high heat. Add peas and carrot and reduce heat to a simmer. Cook for 2 minutes and add asparagus, spinach and seasonings. Cook for 5 minutes, or until vegetables are tender. Increase heat and add chicken.

In small bowl, combine cornstarch with cold water and mix until thoroughly blended. Add to the hot soup, stirring until slightly thickened. Remove from heat and stir in chives just before serving.

*Serves 4*

# Chicken Stir-Fry

*Chicken and fried rice makes a quick one-dish meal. Use gluten-free tamari sauce if you cannot find gluten-free soy sauce. Use broccoli instead of celery to add more nutrition, if you prefer.*

- ½ onion, sliced and quartered
- 1 tablespoon canola oil
- 1 stalk celery, sliced diagonally
- 1 clove garlic, minced
- 1 tablespoon gluten-free soy sauce
- 1 cup cold, cooked rice
- ½ cup cooked chicken, cubed

Heat a wok or large nonstick skillet over medium-high heat. Add oil, then cook onion, celery and garlic, stirring constantly, for 1 minute. Add soy sauce and stir well.

Add rice and chicken, stirring to break up and color rice evenly.

Cook until heated through and serve.

*Serves 2*

## Quick Fish Florentine

*Spinach is a classic accompaniment to fish. This quick and easy recipe has no flour or breadcrumbs. Serve with rice or potatoes.*

- 1 cup spinach, cooked
- 2 (6-ounce) flounder filets, fresh or frozen and defrosted
- 2 tablespoons butter, melted
- Salt and pepper, to taste
- 1 teaspoon fresh lemon juice
- 1 teaspoon lemon zest

Make two beds of spinach on a microwave-safe baking dish. Coat fish with butter on both sides and season with salt and pepper.

Place fish on top of the spinach and microwave on high for 3 to 5 minutes, until fish is opaque and flakes easily.

Drizzle the fish with lemon juice and sprinkle with zest before serving.

*Serves 2*

# White Chili

*This mild chicken chili is perfect for potlucks and parties. Use any kind of white beans you like, such as great northern or cannellini beans. Top each serving with chopped fresh cilantro, green onions and shredded cheese.*

- 1 tablespoon olive oil
- 1 pound boneless, skinless chicken breasts or thighs, cut into 1-inch cubes
- 1 onion, chopped
- 2 (15 ½-ounce) cans white beans, rinsed and drained
- 1 (14 ½-ounce) can chicken broth
- 2 (4-ounce) cans green chilies, chopped
- 2 cloves garlic, minced
- ½ teaspoon salt
- 1 teaspoon ground cumin
- 1 teaspoon dried oregano
- ½ cup light sour cream
- Salt and freshly ground pepper, to taste

In a large Dutch oven, sauté the chicken and onion in oil for 5 minutes over medium-high heat.

Add the beans, broth, green chilies, garlic, salt and spices. Bring to a boil, then lower the heat and simmer for 20 minutes.

Remove from heat and mix in the sour cream. Season with salt and pepper to taste.

*Serves 4*

## Pasta Primavera

*Pasta primavera means "spring pasta" in Italian. Fresh, colorful vegetables are tossed with gluten-free pasta in this easy-to-make entrée. Enjoy this meal with a glass of white wine.*

- 2 tablespoons extra virgin olive oil
- 1 clove garlic, minced
- 1 bunch asparagus, trimmed and cut into 1-inch pieces
- 1 sweet red pepper, diced
- 2 cups fresh spinach
- 1 (14 ½-ounce) can diced tomatoes, drained
- 8 ounces gluten-free spaghetti, cooked according to package directions
- ½ cup fresh parsley, chopped
- ½ cup Parmesan cheese, grated

Heat a large nonstick skillet over medium heat. Add oil and garlic and cook for 30 seconds. Add asparagus and red pepper and sauté for 5 minutes.

Add spinach and tomatoes and cook until spinach is wilted.

Serve vegetables over cooked pasta. Sprinkle with parsley and Parmesan cheese.

*Serves 4*

# Turkey Tetrazzini

*This all-American dish is a great way to use leftover Thanksgiving turkey. Gluten-free pasta and cornstarch as a thickener instead of flour are the only adjustments to this classic recipe. Serve with a green salad.*

- Nonstick cooking spray
- 2 tablespoons unsalted butter
- 1 cup fresh mushrooms, sliced
- ½ cup onion, minced
- 1 stalk celery, sliced thin
- 1 clove garlic, minced
- 3 tablespoons cornstarch
- 1 (14 ½-ounce) can chicken broth, divided
- 1 (12-ounce) can evaporated milk
- ½ pound gluten-free spaghetti, cooked according to package directions
- 3 cups cubed cooked turkey (see recipe for Roast Turkey Breast With Pan Gravy)
- ½ teaspoon salt
- ½ teaspoon pepper
- ¼ cup Parmesan cheese, grated
- ½ teaspoon paprika

Preheat oven to 350 degrees. Coat a large casserole dish with nonstick cooking spray.

Heat a large skillet over medium heat, add butter, then cook mushrooms, onion, celery and garlic until tender.

In a small bowl, whisk together cornstarch and ½ cup broth until smooth. Add cornstarch mixture and remaining broth to the pan and bring to a boil. Cook and stir for 2 minutes until thickened. Reduce heat to low and add milk. Cook, stirring for 2 minutes. Stir in the spaghetti, turkey, salt and pepper and mix well.

Transfer to the prepared casserole dish. Cover with foil and bake for 20 minutes. Uncover, sprinkle with Parmesan cheese and paprika, and bake for another 10 minutes until heated through.

*Serves 4*

## Pepper Steak

*This easy stir-fry is perfect for weeknight dinners. Cornstarch is a thickener used in many Asian-style dishes. Add more or less cayenne according to your taste.*

- ½ pound round steak
- 1 tablespoon canola oil
- 1 onion, sliced
- 1 red pepper, sliced
- 1 green pepper, sliced
- 2 cloves garlic, minced
- 1 tablespoon cornstarch
- ¼ cup beef broth
- 2 tablespoons gluten-free soy sauce
- ½ teaspoon salt
- ¼ teaspoon cayenne pepper
- 2 cups hot, cooked rice

Freeze steak for 20 minutes, then slice into very thin strips cutting across the grain, and set aside.

Heat a large frying pan over medium-high heat, add the oil and cook the onion, peppers and garlic for 3 minutes.

In a small bowl, stir cornstarch into broth until smooth.

Add meat to hot pan and cook, stirring frequently, for 2 minutes. Add soy sauce, salt, cayenne and cornstarch broth mixture. Stir constantly until sauce thickens.

Serve over hot rice.

*Serves 4*

# Tuscan Bean Soup

*White beans and kale, staples in Tuscany, are featured in this hearty soup. Beans provide a good source of fiber in a gluten-free diet. Serve the soup with a gluten-free version of focaccia or French bread.*

- 2 tablespoons olive oil
- 1 onion, chopped
- 3 carrots, peeled and sliced thin
- 2 stalks celery, sliced thin
- 3 cloves garlic, minced
- ½ teaspoon salt
- 2 (32-ounce) cartons chicken broth
- 2 (15 ½-ounce) can cannellini beans, rinsed and drained
- ¼ teaspoon dried thyme
- ¼ teaspoon dried sage
- ¼ teaspoon oregano
- 1 bunch kale, stemmed and chopped

Heat a large pot over medium heat and add olive oil. Cook the onion, carrots, celery, garlic and salt over medium-high heat until onions are translucent.

Add broth, beans, thyme, sage and oregano. Stir well and simmer for 20 minutes.

Stir in kale and simmer until wilted.

*Serves 4*

## Baked Lemon Chicken Thighs

*Lemon roast chicken is delicious hot, but also good the next day sliced and added to a salad or sandwich. This easy recipe contains no gluten-free substitutes and would make a fine dish for company. Serve with rice or potatoes and a fresh green vegetable for a meal no one will realize is gluten-free.*

- 2 tablespoons butter, melted
- 2 tablespoons lemon juice
- 1 clove garlic, mashed
- ½ teaspoon salt
- ¼ teaspoon pepper
- 6 boneless, skinless chicken thighs
- ½ teaspoon paprika

Preheat oven to 350 degrees. Grease the baking dish.

Combine butter, lemon juice, garlic, salt and pepper in a small bowl. Arrange chicken thighs in baking dish (leave at least an inch between pieces) and brush with butter mixture.

Sprinkle with paprika, transfer to the oven and bake for 25 to 30 minutes, or until internal temperature reaches 165 degrees.

*Serves 4*

# Chicken With Confetti Rice

*Colorful vegetables add flair to this chicken and rice dish. Rice dishes are a good gluten-free meal option. Swap out asparagus for the broccoli and red peppers for the carrot, if you prefer.*

- ½ cup chicken broth
- ½ cup broccoli, chopped
- 2 cups cold, cooked rice
- 1 cup cooked chicken, shredded
- 1 grated carrot
- 2 scallions, sliced thin, white and green parts separated
- ½ teaspoon salt
- ¼ teaspoon pepper
- 2 tablespoons fresh parsley, minced

Bring chicken broth to a simmer over medium heat in a large skillet. Add broccoli and cook 2 minutes. Add rice, chicken, carrot, white part of scallions, salt and pepper.

Stir to break up rice, cover and cook over low heat until heated through.

Garnish with parsley and green tops of scallions.

*Serves 2*

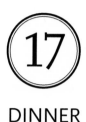

# DINNER

## Alfredo Sauce

*This sauce is classically served on fettuccine. No flour is needed for thickening; it's rich with cream and cheese. Use it on pizza, pasta or to top potatoes or vegetables such as cauliflower or broccoli.*

- ¼ cup unsalted butter
- 1 cup cream
- 1 cup Parmesan cheese, grated
- Freshly ground black pepper

Melt butter in a saucepan over medium-low heat and add cream. Heat over low heat for 5 minutes, stirring constantly. Add cheese and pepper and whisk until smooth.

*Makes about 1 ½ cups*

## Roasted Vegetable Pizza With Alfredo Sauce

*This vegetable pizza will satisfy the craving for a food most everyone loves. Experiment with different combinations of roasted vegetables. Serve with wine and a green salad.*

- 1 bunch asparagus, washed and trimmed, cut into 3-inch pieces
- 1 red onion, sliced into half rounds
- 1 red pepper, cored and sliced
- 1 cup mushrooms, sliced
- 1 small eggplant, ends trimmed, cut into quarter rounds
- 2 tablespoons olive oil
- 1 Pizza Crust
- 1 recipe Alfredo Sauce
- ½ cup mozzarella cheese, grated
- 1 teaspoon Italian herb blend

Preheat oven to 400 degrees.

Arrange vegetables in 1 or 2 roasting pans, to accommodate a single layer. Drizzle with olive oil and toss until evenly coated. Arrange in single layer and transfer to the oven. Roast for 15 to 20 minutes or until tender. Remove from oven.

Spread Alfredo Sauce over Pizza Crust in a thin layer. Arrange roasted vegetables and sprinkle evenly with mozzarella and herbs. (Do not overload the pizza. There will be leftover vegetables and sauce. They can be stored in the refrigerator and used later on sandwiches, salads or pasta.)

Bake pizza for 5 to 10 minutes, until cheese is melted and crust is crisp.

*Serves 4*

## Pasta Carbonara

*Eggs, cheese and a bit of pasta water form the thick and creamy sauce for this pasta. The name carbonara (Italian for "charcoal kiln") comes from the flecks of black pepper. Serve with a green salad.*

- 12 ounces gluten-free penne pasta
- 6 slices bacon, diced
- 2 eggs
- ¾ cup pecorino romano cheese, grated
- Freshly ground black pepper

Cook pasta according to package directions. Drain pasta and reserve 1 cup of cooking water.

While the pasta is cooking, in a large skillet over medium heat, cook the bacon until crisp and drain on paper towels. Pour out bacon fat, but reserve the pan. In a medium bowl, whisk together the eggs and cheese.

Place the drained pasta in the skillet, and add the eggs and cheese mixture. Toss the hot pasta with the sauce off the heat, stirring constantly, until the eggs begin to thicken. Add reserved pasta water as necessary to bring sauce to the desired thickness.

Continue tossing until all the pasta is evenly coated, then stir in bacon. Season with plenty of pepper and serve.

*Serves 4*

# Lo Mein

*This Chinese dish combines noodles and stir-fry. Use gluten-free rice noodles or any other gluten-free noodles you like. This dish can also be made with chicken or pork instead of shrimp.*

- ½ pound raw shrimp, shelled and deveined
- 2 teaspoons dry sherry
- 1 teaspoon cornstarch
- ½ pound gluten-free rice noodles
- 1 teaspoon toasted sesame oil
- ¼ cup chicken broth
- 2 tablespoons gluten-free soy sauce
- ½ teaspoon sugar
- 2 tablespoons canola oil, divided
- 2 teaspoons fresh ginger, grated
- 1 small onion, sliced in thin wedges
- ½ cup cabbage, shredded
- 1 red bell pepper, cored and sliced in strips

Combine the shrimp, sherry and cornstarch in a small bowl and marinate for 15 minutes.

Cook noodles according to package directions until al dente. Drain well, rinse with cold water and drain again. Toss noodles with the sesame oil.

Combine broth, soy sauce and sugar in a small bowl and set aside.

Heat a wok or large frying pan over medium high heat and add a tablespoon of oil. When oil is hot, add ginger and stir-fry for 30 seconds. Add shrimp and stir-fry until they turn pink. Remove from wok.

Add the second tablespoon of oil and, when hot, add the onion. Stir-fry for a minute, then add the cabbage and stir-fry for another minute. Add the pepper, stir-fry for another minute and remove from the pan. Add the noodles and sauce to the pan.

Reduce heat to medium and let the noodles absorb the sauce. Add the shrimp and vegetables back into the pan. Heat through and serve.

*Serves 2*

# Battered Fish or Shrimp

*Fish and chips is something you can make from scratch at home. Rice flour creates a very crunchy coating. Serve with oven-roasted potato wedges or French fries.*

- 1 cup rice flour
- 1 teaspoon salt
- ½ teaspoon pepper
- ½ teaspoon paprika
- ¾ cup water
- 2 eggs, separated

- 2 teaspoons extra virgin olive oil
- ¼ cup canola oil
- 8 skinless fish fillets, about 3 ounces each, or 1 pound large shrimp, peeled, deveined and patted dry

In a large, shallow bowl, mix flour, salt, pepper and paprika.

In a small bowl, whisk together water, egg yolks and olive oil. Stir into the flour mixture.

In another bowl, beat the egg whites until firm peaks form. Fold into the batter.

Heat canola oil in a large skillet over medium-high heat. Dip fillets or shrimp into batter, one at a time, and shake off excess batter.

Fry fish in batches 4 to 5 minutes per side (cook shrimp for 2 minutes on each side). Add more oil and adjust heat if necessary between batches.

*Serves 4*

# Beef Stroganoff

*This rich Russian beef dish is creamy and comforting. Rice flour thickens the sauce, replacing wheat flour. Use light sour cream if you want to decrease the calories in this dish.*

- 1 pound beef sirloin
- 3 tablespoons rice flour, divided
- ½ teaspoon salt
- ½ teaspoon fresh ground black pepper
- 2 tablespoons canola oil, divided
- ½ cup fresh mushrooms, sliced
- 1 onion, chopped
- 2 cloves garlic, minced
- 1 tablespoon gluten-free ketchup
- 1 (14 ½-ounce) can beef broth
- 1 cup sour cream
- 3 tablespoons dry white wine
- 16 ounces gluten-free noodles, cooked according to package directions
- Butter to dress noodles

Freeze beef for 20 minutes, then cut into ¼-inch slices, across the grain. In a medium bowl, toss the slices of beef with 1 tablespoon rice flour, salt and pepper.

Heat a large skillet over medium heat and add 1 tablespoon oil. Add beef and stir-fry quickly until just barely cooked. Add mushrooms, onions and garlic and cook for 4 minutes. Transfer meat and vegetables to a large bowl and set aside.

Add the remaining oil to the pan and blend in remaining rice flour. Add the ketchup and beef broth and blend with a spoon. Cook over medium heat, stirring constantly, until sauce is thickened. Return meat mixture to pan. Stir in sour cream and wine. Cook over low heat until hot, but do not boil.

Serve over hot, buttered noodles.

*Serves 4*

# Roast Turkey Breast With Pan Gravy

*Roast turkey with homemade gravy is a Thanksgiving classic. You can enjoy gravy when it's made with rice flour or cornstarch as a thickener instead of wheat flour.*

- Boneless turkey breast, 4 to 5 pounds
- 2 tablespoons melted butter
- Salt and pepper, to taste
- 2 (14-ounce) cans chicken broth, divided
- 3 tablespoons rice flour

Preheat oven to 450 degrees.

Pat turkey dry with paper towels and place on rack in a roasting pan. Brush with melted butter and season generously with salt and pepper.

Transfer to the oven and roast for 45 minutes to 1 hour, basting twice with ¼ cup broth. When an instant-read thermometer registers 155 degrees, remove the turkey from the oven. Set on a platter and tent loosely with foil. Turkey should rest for 10 minutes before being carved.

Remove as much fat from roasting pan as possible, leaving drippings and any brown bits. Deglaze pan over medium heat with the remainder of the chicken broth.

In a small mixing bowl, mix rice flour with enough water to make a thin paste. Bring broth to a boil and pour in the rice flour paste, stirring constantly until gravy thickens. Adjust salt and pepper to taste.

*Serves 6–8*

## Roast Chicken

*Roast chicken is a crowd pleaser. The pan drippings can be easily turned into a gluten-free gravy with broth and cornstarch or rice flour (see Roast Turkey Breast With Pan Gravy for gravy ideas). Serve with roasted potatoes and a green vegetable.*

- 1 broiler or fryer chicken, about 3 pounds
- Salt and pepper, to taste
- 1 onion, quartered
- 1 stalk celery, chopped
- 1 clove garlic, crushed
- Olive oil

Preheat oven to 350 degrees.

Wash and pat dry the chicken and place on a rack in roasting pan. Sprinkle cavity with salt and pepper. Put onion, celery and garlic in cavity. Rub chicken with olive oil and transfer to the oven.

Roast for 1 to 1 ¼ hours, or until a meat thermometer inserted into the thickest part of the thigh reads 165 degrees.

Let stand 10 minutes before carving. Discard vegetables in cavity.

*Serves 4*

# Meat Loaf

*Meat loaf is an American classic. Serve with mashed potatoes and a vegetable side dish such as carrots or spinach. Store leftovers in the refrigerator up to three days.*

- 2 egg whites
- 3 slices stale gluten-free bread
- ½ cup milk
- ½ cup onion, finely chopped
- ½ teaspoon dry mustard
- 1 teaspoon dried parsley flakes
- 1 teaspoon garlic salt
- ½ teaspoon ground black pepper
- 1 pound lean ground beef
- Nonstick cooking spray
- 3 tablespoons gluten-free ketchup

Preheat oven to 350 degrees. Spray an 11 x 7-inch loaf pan sprayed with nonstick cooking spray.

Beat the egg whites in a large bowl. Set aside.

Crumble bread and add to another large mixing bowl with the milk. Let stand for 5 minutes. Stir in the onion and seasonings, crumble the beef into the bowl, then the reserved egg whites, and mix well.

Form into a loaf and place in the center of prepared loaf pan. Transfer to the oven and bake for 35 minutes.

Drain off pan juices. Spoon ketchup over the top and return to oven for 15 minutes or until meat thermometer reads 160 degrees.

Let rest at least 10 minutes before slicing.

*Serves 4*

# Cheesy Risotto

*This cheddar rice dish will help satisfy the craving for macaroni and cheese. For more cheesy flavor, top with a sprinkling of grated Parmesan cheese. Serve with a green salad.*

- 2 tablespoons unsalted butter
- ½ cup onion, finely chopped
- 1 ½ cups short-grain rice, such as Arborio
- 4 cups hot chicken or vegetable broth, divided
- ¼ teaspoon dry mustard
- 1 cup cheddar cheese, grated
- 2 tablespoons fresh parsley, chopped

Melt the butter in a medium saucepan over medium heat and cook the onion until transparent. Add the rice and cook, stirring, for 2 minutes.

Turn up the heat and add 1 cup broth and the mustard. Stir until rice absorbs the broth. Continue adding the broth 1 cup at a time and stirring until absorbed. Cook on very low heat until the rice is al dente, about 18 to 20 minutes.

Turn the heat off, then add the cheese and stir into the rice until it melts. Serve garnished with parsley.

*Serves 4*

# Beef and Bean Tacos

*Crisp corn tacos are a gluten-free treat. If you can find Mexican cheese, such as cotija or queso fresco, feel free to use that instead of the Monterey Jack or cheddar. Serve with guacamole and carrot and celery sticks for dipping.*

- 1 pound lean ground beef
- ½ cup onion, chopped
- 1 clove garlic, minced
- 1 teaspoon chili powder
- ½ teaspoon dried oregano
- 1 (12-ounce) can black beans, rinsed and drained
- 1 (4-ounce) can green chilies, chopped
- 12 gluten-free taco shells (100 percent corn)
- 1 cup Monterey Jack or cheddar cheese, grated
- ½ cup lettuce, shredded
- ½ cup chunky tomato salsa

Heat a large frying pan over medium-high heat.

Cook ground beef, onion, garlic, chili powder and oregano for 5 to 7 minutes. Break meat up well with a spatula as it cooks.

Add the beans and chilies to the pan and smash the beans with the back of a wooden spoon. Stir well and heat through. If the pan is too dry, add a tablespoon of salsa liquid.

Warm taco shells according to package directions. Fill shells with meat mixture, leaving room to top with cheese and lettuce. Serve with salsa.

*Serves 6*

## Chicken Fried Rice for One

*This hearty stir-fried rice dish is a good way to use up leftover rice and chicken. Cold rice is best for stir-fry dishes because the starch enables the rice to stay firm. Substitute gluten-free tamari if you cannot find gluten-free soy sauce.*

- 1 teaspoon canola oil
- 1 carrot, thinly sliced
- ¼ cup onions, slivered
- ½ cup cooked chicken, shredded
- ¼ cup frozen peas
- 1 tablespoon gluten-free soy sauce
- 1 cup cold, cooked rice
- A few drops toasted sesame oil
- ¼ teaspoon red pepper flakes

Heat a medium frying pan over medium heat, add the oil and cook the carrots for 1 minute. Add the onion and stir-fry for 2 minutes. Add chicken, peas and soy sauce, and continue stir-frying for another minute.

Crumble the rice into the pan, separating it into individual grains. Cook, stirring, until heated through.

Sprinkle with sesame oil and red pepper and serve.

*Serves 1*

## Quick Enchiladas for One

*Corn tortillas dipped in sauce and filled with meat or cheese make luscious enchiladas. Carefully read the labels of prepackaged shredded cheeses, which may contain wheat flour to keep the cheese from clumping. Serve with rice and beans.*

- 2 corn tortillas
- ½ cup green or red enchilada sauce, divided
- ½ cup cooked chicken or turkey, shredded
- 1 scallion, sliced thin
- ½ cup cheddar or Monterey Jack cheese, shredded

Wrap the tortillas in paper towels and warm them in the microwave for 15 to 20 seconds to make them pliable.

Spread 2 tablespoons of enchilada sauce on each tortilla. Place half the chicken and scallions on each tortilla and roll to form an enchilada. Place each enchilada, seam side down, in a small microwave-safe casserole dish with a lid. Cover enchiladas with the remaining sauce and sprinkle with cheese.

Cover the dish, then microwave the enchiladas at 50 percent power for 5 minutes, or until cheese is melted and enchiladas are heated through.

*Serves 1*

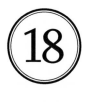

# DESSERT

## Refrigerator Cookies

*Refrigerator cookies are ready when you are. Rice and soy flour have a mild flavor and help approximate all-purpose wheat flour in this recipe. Swap out walnuts or almonds for the pecans, if you prefer.*

- 1 ½ cups dark brown sugar
- 1 stick butter or margarine
- 1 egg
- ¾ cup soy flour
- ¼ cup rice flour
- 1 teaspoon cinnamon
- ½ cup chopped pecans

Cream the sugar and butter in a large mixing bowl using a wooden spoon. When light and fluffy, beat in the egg, then the flours and cinnamon. Mix the chopped nuts into the dough. Form the dough into a roll 6 inches long 1 ½ inches in diameter. Wrap tightly in plastic wrap and refrigerate for at least 1 hour, or up to 1 month.

When ready to bake, preheat oven to 375 degrees and grease a large cookie sheet.

Unwrap cookie dough and slice ¼-inch thick slices. Place on cookie sheet and bake at 375 degrees for 10 to 12 minutes. Transfer to a rack to cool.

*Makes 2 dozen*

# Gluten-Free Snickerdoodles

*Snickerdoodles are cinnamon sugar cookies that are crunchy on the outside yet gooey on the inside. Potato starch, cornstarch and tapioca flour help to create the right texture. Serve with hot or iced tea.*

## Cookies

- 1 ½ cups sugar
- 1 cup (2 sticks) butter
- 4 egg yolks
- 1 teaspoon vanilla
- 1 ½ cups potato starch (also known as potato starch flour)
- ⅔ cup tapioca flour

- ⅓ cup cornstarch
- 2 teaspoons baking powder
- 1 teaspoon salt

## Cinnamon sugar dip

- 2 tablespoons sugar
- 2 teaspoons cinnamon

Preheat oven to 375 degrees and grease a large cookie sheet.

## Cookies

In a large bowl, cream the sugar and butter until light and fluffy. Blend the egg yolks and vanilla into the creamed mixture.

In a separate bowl, combine flours, baking powder and salt then stir into butter mixture. Work the dough until you can form small balls.

## Cinnamon sugar dip

In a small dish, mix together the sugar and cinnamon.

Roll rounded teaspoons of dough into balls, roll in cinnamon sugar, and place 2 inches apart on prepared cookie sheet.

Bake for 8 to 10 minutes. Transfer to a rack to cool. Store in an airtight container for up to 3 days.

*Makes 2 dozen*

# Creamy Rice Pudding

*Luscious rice pudding is a creamy treat. Naturally gluten-free, rice pudding relies on eggs and the starch from the rice as thickeners. Serve with fresh berries.*

- 4 cups whole milk
- 2 eggs, beaten
- ½ cup sugar
- ½ cup uncooked short-grain white rice
- ½ cup golden raisins (optional)
- 1 tablespoon butter
- 1 teaspoon vanilla extract
- ½ teaspoon cinnamon
- Pinch of nutmeg

Preheat oven to 300 degrees. Grease a 2-quart baking dish.

Combine the milk and eggs in a large mixing bowl and beat together. Stir in the sugar, rice, raisins, butter, vanilla, cinnamon and nutmeg.

Pour into prepared dish and cover loosely with foil. Transfer to the oven and bake for 2 hours, or until thick and creamy. Stir every 15 minutes during the first hour.

*Serves 6–8*

# Angel Food Cake With Lemon Zest Glaze

*Angel food cake is light and airy. The delicate, tender texture comes from a combination of potato starch and cornstarch, rather than cake flour. Top with a zesty lemon glaze, and serve with fresh berries.*

### Cake

- ½ cup powdered sugar
- ½ cup potato starch (also known as potato starch flour)
- ¼ cup cornstarch
- ½ cup granulated sugar
- ¾ cup egg whites (from 7 eggs), at room temperature
- ¾ teaspoon cream of tartar
- ¼ teaspoon salt
- 1 teaspoon vanilla or almond extract

### Glaze

- 2 to 3 tablespoons milk
- 1 cup confectioners' sugar
- ½ teaspoon lemon zest

Preheat oven to 375 degrees. Set aside an ungreased 9-inch tube pan.

### Cake

Sift together the powdered sugar, potato starch and cornstarch into a medium bowl.

Measure granulated sugar into a small bowl.

In a large glass or metal bowl, combine the egg whites, cream of tartar and salt. With an electric mixer, beat the egg white mixture on high until well blended. Continue beating and gradually add the granulated sugar. Beat until sugar dissolves and soft peaks form.

Gently fold the vanilla and a quarter of the flour mixture into the egg whites. Continue folding in a quarter of the flour mixture at a time until it all disappears into the egg whites.

Pour batter into the tube pan and cut through a few times with a knife to break up any large air bubbles. Transfer to the oven and bake for 35 minutes, until the top springs back when touched lightly.

Remove from oven and invert the pan onto a bottle or a heatproof funnel, so the tube points down, to cool. Cake must be completely cool before removing from pan.

## Glaze

In a small mixing bowl, mix 2 tablespoons milk into the powdered sugar. Add more milk, a teaspoon at a time, to reach the desired consistency. Stir in lemon zest.

When the cake is cool, drizzle with glaze.

*Serves 8*

## Peanut Butter Cookies

*Nutty peanut butter cookies are protein-packed. No flour is necessary for this recipe. Serve with milk or coffee.*

- 2 cups crunchy peanut butter
- 2 cups sugar
- 4 eggs, beaten
- ½ teaspoon cinnamon

Preheat oven to 350 degrees. Grease a large cookie sheet.

Combine the peanut butter, sugar, eggs and cinnamon in a large bowl and mix until smooth.

Drop by spoonfuls onto the greased cookie sheet. Transfer to the oven and bake for 10 to 12 minutes until lightly browned.

Cool completely on the cookie sheet before transferring to a rack.

*Makes 2 dozen*

# Crumb Crust

*A crumb crust is crisp but not flaky. Brown rice flour and ground almonds give this crust a nutty, crunchy texture. Use this crust with pudding-type fillings, such as the Kahlua Cream Pie Filling or Banana Cream Pie Filling.*

- Nonstick cooking spray
- 1 cup brown rice flour
- ½ cup almonds, ground
- ½ teaspoon cinnamon
- 3 tablespoons apple juice concentrate, thawed
- 2 tablespoons canola oil

Preheat oven to 375 degrees. Spray a 9-inch pie pan with nonstick cooking spray.

Combine the rice flour, almonds, cinnamon, apple juice concentrate and canola oil in a bowl. Press mixture into the bottom and up the sides of prepared pie plate.

Bake at 375 degrees for 10 to 14 minutes. Cool before filling.

*Makes 1 crust*

## Kahlua Cream Pie Filling

*Coffee liqueur and a creamy filling make a sophisticated dessert. Cream cheese and condensed milk form the custard-like filling of this pie. Top with fresh raspberries, if desired, and serve with coffee.*

- 2 teaspoons unflavored gelatin
- ¼ cup cold water
- 12 ounces cream cheese, softened
- 2 tablespoons sugar
- ¾ cup sweetened condensed milk
- ¼ cup Kahlua or other coffee liqueur
- 2 cups whipped cream
- 1 Crumb Crust

In a small saucepan, sprinkle gelatin over cold water and let stand for 1 minute. Heat mixture over low heat, stirring constantly, until gelatin is completely dissolved. Remove from heat.

In a large bowl, beat together cream cheese and sugar until smooth. Add gelatin mixture, condensed milk and Kahlua. Beat until well blended. Gently fold in whipped cream. Pour into Crumb Crust.

Refrigerate, covered, for 4 hours until set.

*Serves 8*

# Banana Cream Pie Filling

*This creamy pie features a custard filling. Cornstarch and eggs are used to thicken the custard. This pie can easily be made the night before you plan to serve it.*

- 2 tablespoons water
- 1 ½ teaspoons unflavored gelatin
- 1 ¼ cups whole milk
- 3 egg yolks
- ⅓ cup sugar
- 1 ½ tablespoons cornstarch
- 2 ½ teaspoons vanilla extract, divided
- 1 ¾ cups whipping cream, chilled
- ¼ cup confectioners' sugar
- 4 ripe bananas, peeled and thinly sliced
- 1 Crumb Crust

Pour the water into a small bowl and sprinkle with gelatin. Let stand for 10 minutes.

In a medium saucepan, bring milk to a simmer.

Whisk together egg yolks, sugar, cornstarch and 2 teaspoons vanilla until thick. Gradually whisk yolk mixture into hot milk. Cook over medium heat, stirring constantly, until mixture just comes to a boil and thickens.

Remove from heat, add gelatin and stir to dissolve. Place plastic wrap directly onto pudding and chill until cool, about 30 minutes.

Beat cream, confectioners' sugar and ½ teaspoon vanilla in a large bowl until it forms stiff peaks. Gently fold 1 ½ cups cream into pudding. Fold in bananas and spoon into Crumb Crust. Cover filling completely with remaining whipped cream.

Chill for 3 to 6 hours before serving.

*Serves 6–8*

## Carrot Cake

*Mayonnaise is the unexpected addition to this carrot cake, helping to add moisture. A combination of rice flour, potato starch and soy flour give the cake structure and a tender crumb. Serve with coffee or tea.*

- Nonstick cooking spray
- 2 (12-ounce) cans unsweetened crushed pineapple, drained
- 1 ½ cups sugar
- 4 eggs
- ¾ cup mayonnaise
- 1 ½ cups rice flour
- ½ cup potato starch (also known as potato starch flour)
- ½ cup soy flour
- 2 teaspoons baking soda
- 2 teaspoons cinnamon
- 1 teaspoon xanthan gum
- ½ teaspoon powdered ginger
- ½ teaspoon salt
- 3 ¼ cups carrots, grated
- 1 cup walnuts, chopped

Preheat oven to 350 degrees. Spray a 13 x 9-inch pan with nonstick cooking spray.

In a large mixing bowl, mix the pineapple, sugar, eggs and mayonnaise until completely blended.

Combine the flours, starch, baking soda, cinnamon, xanthan gum, ginger and salt. Gradually add to the sugar mixture, beating well between each addition, until well mixed. Stir in the carrots and nuts.

Pour into prepared pan and bake for 40 to 50 minutes, until a cake tester or a toothpick inserted in the center comes out clean. Cool completely on a rack before frosting with Cream Cheese Frosting.

*Serves 18*

## Cream Cheese Frosting

*Cream Cheese Frosting is the traditional choice for Carrot Cake. This frosting can also be used on cupcakes. Add more vanilla or lemon extract, if you'd like.*

- 4 ounces cream cheese, softened
- ¼ cup butter, softened
- 2 ½ cups confectioners' sugar
- 1 teaspoon lemon zest
- ½ teaspoon pure vanilla extract

Beat cream cheese and butter in a mixing bowl until fluffy.

Add sugar, lemon zest and vanilla and beat until smooth.

Spread over cooled Carrot Cake.

*Makes enough frosting for 1 Carrot Cake*

# Spice Cake

*A spice cake is perfect for entertaining or potlucks. A combination of brown rice flour and soy flour gives the cake structure. If you like, you can frost this cake with a very thin layer of Cream Cheese Frosting or simply dust it with confectioners' sugar. Serve with coffee or tea.*

- ¾ cup unsweetened applesauce
- ½ cup honey
- 2 eggs
- 2 tablespoons canola oil
- 1 teaspoon pure vanilla extract
- 1 cup brown rice flour
- ½ cup soy flour
- 2 teaspoons powdered ginger
- 2 teaspoons cinnamon
- ¼ teaspoon ground nutmeg
- ¼ teaspoon allspice
- Pinch of ground cloves
- 1 ¼ teaspoons baking powder
- ½ teaspoon salt
- ¼ teaspoon baking soda
- ¾ cup walnuts, chopped

Preheat oven to 350 degrees. Grease an 8-inch square baking pan.

In a large bowl, beat the applesauce, honey, eggs, oil and vanilla until completely blended.

Combine the flours, spices, baking powder, salt and baking soda in another mixing bowl and mix well. Gradually beat the flour into the applesauce mixture until combined. Fold in the walnuts.

Pour batter into prepared pan, transfer to the oven and bake for 30 to 34 minutes, or until a cake tester or a toothpick inserted in the center comes out clean. Cool completely on a wire rack.

*Serves 10–12*

# Apple Crisp

*Apple crisp is a favorite autumn dessert. Rice flour and tapioca flour give this dessert its signature crunchy topping. Serve warm with vanilla ice cream.*

- Nonstick cooking spray
- 6 Granny Smith apples, peeled, cored and sliced
- 2 teaspoons cinnamon
- ½ cup brown sugar, divided
- ¼ cup rice flour
- ¼ cup tapioca flour
- ½ cup walnuts, chopped
- ¼ cup butter
- Vanilla ice cream (optional)

Preheat oven to 375 degrees. Spray a deep-dish pie plate with nonstick cooking spray.

Pile apples slices into the pie plate. In a small bowl, mix together cinnamon and ¼ cup brown sugar and sprinkle evenly over the apples.

Combine the flours, nuts and the rest of the sugar in a bowl. Add the butter and knead until mixture resembles breadcrumbs. Spread evenly over apples.

Transfer to the oven and bake for 25 minutes, until apples are tender and crumb topping is golden. Allow to cool 10 minutes before serving.

*Serves 8–10*

## Tropical Sorbet

*Fresh fruit is the basis for this very refreshing sorbet. It can also be served as a palate cleanser between courses. Substitute tangerine juice for the orange juice, for a more exotic flavor.*

- 2 cups fresh pineapple, cut into 2-inch pieces
- 2 cups fresh mango, sliced
- 2 tablespoons sugar
- 2 tablespoons orange juice

Line a jelly roll pan with plastic wrap. Arrange fruit in 1 layer. Cover and seal with more plastic wrap and freeze overnight.

Transfer frozen fruit to the food processor and pulse until finely chopped. Add sugar and orange juice and process for 30 seconds.

Taste and add more sugar if necessary. Blend for 5 minutes or until very smooth, scraping down the sides a few times.

Spoon into a tightly covered container and return to freezer. Transfer to the refrigerator for 20 minutes before scooping and serving.

*Serves 4*

## Microwave Pudding

*This easy, dairy-free pudding is creamy and rich, thickened with cornstarch. Zest the lemon before squeezing it. Serve topped with fresh fruit.*

- 1 cup sugar
- 6 tablespoons cornstarch
- 1 tablespoon lemon zest, finely grated
- Pinch of salt
- 4 ¼ cups almond milk, divided
- Juice of 2 lemons, divided

In a large microwave-safe bowl, mix the sugar, cornstarch, lemon zest and salt. Slowly mix in ⅓ cup almond milk to make a smooth paste. Gradually whisk in the rest of the milk, keeping the mixture smooth.

Transfer the bowl to the microwave and cook on high for 2 minutes. Stir well. Continue cooking for 2 more minutes, whisk, and cook again. Repeat until the mixture thickens.

Add half the lemon juice and mix well. Taste and add as much of the rest of the juice as you like. Place plastic wrap directly on the pudding and chill in the refrigerator until firm.

*Serves 4*

# TOP TEN GLUTEN-FREE RECIPES FOR AMERICA'S FAVORITE FOODS

## Chocolate Chip Cookies

*A truly original American recipe, the smell of chocolate chip cookies baking is almost as delicious as the taste. A combination of soy and rice flour replaces wheat flour.*

- 1 cup (2 sticks) butter or margarine
- 1 cup light brown sugar
- 2 eggs
- 1 teaspoon vanilla extract
- 2 cups soy flour

- ¼ cup rice flour
- 1 teaspoon baking soda
- ½ teaspoon salt
- ½ teaspoon cinnamon
- 1 (12-ounce) package semisweet chocolate chips

Preheat oven to 350 degrees.

In a large mixing bowl, cream the butter, brown sugar, eggs and vanilla with an electric mixer. Combine the flours, baking soda, salt and cinnamon in a separate mixing bowl, then add to the creamed butter mixture and mix well. Stir in the chips.

Drop by teaspoonfuls onto ungreased cookie sheets. Bake for approximately 10 minutes. Cool on a wire rack.

*Makes 3 dozen*

## Mac and Cheese Casserole

*Nothing quite says comfort like macaroni and cheese. Here, rice flour, gluten-free macaroni and gluten-free breadcrumbs replace more conventional wheat-based ingredients. Look for macaroni made from rice or corn.*

- 1 ½ cups milk, divided
- 2 tablespoons rice flour
- 2 tablespoons butter
- 1 teaspoon onion powder
- 1 teaspoon dried parsley
- ½ teaspoon pepper
- Dash cayenne pepper
- 8 ounces sharp cheddar cheese, cubed
- 2 cups gluten-free elbow macaroni, cooked according to package directions
- ¼ cup gluten-free breadcrumbs
- ¼ cup Parmesan cheese, grated
- 1 teaspoon paprika

Preheat oven to 350 degrees. Lightly grease a 9 x 13-inch baking dish.

In a small bowl, whisk together ¼ cup milk and rice flour into a smooth paste.

In a large saucepan, heat butter and remaining milk almost to a boil. Add rice flour paste and stir until thickened. Add onion powder, parsley and peppers. Stir in cheddar cheese and cook over medium heat until cheese melts. Stir in cooked pasta and mix well.

Pour into baking dish. In a small bowl, combine breadcrumbs, Parmesan cheese and paprika and sprinkle evenly over top of macaroni. Transfer to the oven and bake for 25 minutes, until top is browned.

*Serves 6–8*

## Brownies

*Rich and fudgy brownies will satisfy any chocolate craving. This version uses applesauce to add moisture, and a combination of sorghum flour and tapioca starch. Serve with coffee or cold milk.*

- ¾ cup sugar
- ¼ cup canola oil
- ¼ cup unsweetened applesauce
- 1 teaspoon vanilla extract
- 2 eggs
- ¼ cup sorghum flour
- ¼ cup tapioca starch
- ¼ cup unsweetened cocoa powder
- 1 teaspoon baking powder
- ½ teaspoon salt
- ½ cup semisweet chocolate chips
- ½ cup walnuts, chopped

Preheat oven to 350 degrees. Grease an 8-inch square baking pan.

In a large bowl, combine sugar, oil and applesauce. Add vanilla and beat in eggs, one at a time, until well mixed.

In a separate bowl, mix together the flour, starch, cocoa, baking powder and salt.

Stir flour mixture into egg mixture until just blended, but do not over-mix. Stir in chips and nuts.

Spread batter into the prepared pan and transfer to the oven. Bake for 35 to 40 minutes, or until a toothpick inserted in the center comes out clean.

Cool completely on a wire rack before cutting into squares.

*Makes 2 dozen*

## Blueberry Muffins

*Muffins should be tender, and actually benefit from gluten-free flour. Use fresh blueberries or thawed frozen blueberries. Serve these muffins warm from the oven.*

- ¼ cup sugar
- 2 tablespoons butter or margarine
- 2 eggs
- 1 cup rice flour
- ¼ teaspoon salt
- 2 teaspoons baking powder
- ½ cup milk
- ½ teaspoon vanilla extract
- ¼ cup blueberries

Preheat the oven to 350 degrees. Line 8 muffin cups with paper liners.

With an electric mixer, cream together the sugar and butter in a large mixing bowl. Beat in the eggs.

Sift together the flour, salt and baking powder into a large mixing bowl. Add to the egg mixture about half at a time, alternating with the milk. Do not overbeat.

Stir in the vanilla and blueberries.

Spoon into muffin cups, transfer to the oven and bake for about 20 minutes, or until a toothpick inserted into a muffin comes out clean.

*Makes 8 muffins*

## Pancakes

*Weekend breakfasts are the perfect time to whip up a batch of fresh, made-from-scratch pancakes. A combination of brown rice flour and sorghum flour replaces wheat. Serve with butter, maple syrup or fresh fruit—or all three!*

- ½ cup brown rice flour
- ½ cup sorghum flour
- 1 teaspoon baking powder
- ¼ teaspoon baking soda
- ¼ teaspoon salt
- 1 cup milk
- 1 egg
- 1 tablespoon honey
- 2 teaspoons canola oil, plus more for cooking
- 1 teaspoon pure vanilla extract

In a large mixing bowl, combine flours, baking powder, baking soda and salt.

In another bowl, beat together milk, egg, honey, 2 teaspoons oil and vanilla.

Pour the wet ingredients into the dry ingredients and stir about 1 minute until smooth.

Heat griddle or skillet over medium heat and add a teaspoon of oil.

Measure batter with a ¼ cup measure for each pancake, and pour onto griddle. Cook for 1 to 2 minutes, until bubbles form and edges are cooked. Flip and cook on other side for 1 to 2 minutes until done.

Repeat, remembering to adjust the heat and add more oil between batches as required.

*Makes 8–10 pancakes*

# French Bread

*Crusty baguettes are even better when warm from the oven. Rice flour, tapioca flour and xanthan gum help to replicate the delicate texture of the crumb and crust. Serve fresh French bread at dinner parties or with soups, and use to make sandwiches.*

- 1 ½ teaspoons sugar
- 1 ¾ cups warm water, about 110 degrees
- 2 tablespoons dry active yeast
- 2 cups rice flour
- 1 ¼ cups tapioca flour
- 1 ½ teaspoons salt
- ¾ cup powdered nonfat milk
- 3 ½ teaspoons xanthan gum
- 1 teaspoon cider vinegar
- 4 egg whites, at room temperature

Preheat oven to 400 degrees. Grease 2 French bread pans or 2 cookie sheets.

In a small bowl, add the sugar and warm water to the yeast and set aside for 10 minutes, allowing the yeast to develop.

In the bowl of a stand mixer, combine the flours, salt, powdered milk and xanthan gum. Add the yeast to the flour and blend with the mixer. Add the vinegar and mix. Add the egg whites and beat for 3 minutes.

Transfer the dough to the prepared pans and form loaves. Cut diagonal slashes across the tops of the loaves every 3 inches with a sharp knife. Cover the loaves with clean towels and let rise in a warm place until doubled (about an hour).

Transfer loaves to the oven and bake for 30 minutes.

*Makes 2 loaves*

## Fresh Pasta

*While dried gluten-free pasta is becoming increasingly available, fresh pasta is a great choice to serve company. Potato starch helps the noodles stay pliable. Serve with your favorite pasta sauce.*

- ⅓ cup tapioca flour
- ⅓ cup cornstarch
- 2 tablespoons potato starch (also known as potato starch flour)
- 1 tablespoon xanthan gum
- ½ teaspoon salt
- 2 eggs
- 1 tablespoon olive oil

Combine the tapioca flour, cornstarch, potato starch, xanthan gum and salt in a large mixing bowl.

Beat together eggs and oil in a separate bowl, then pour into flour mixture and stir. Work the dough into a ball and knead for 2 minutes.

Use your pasta machine to form pasta in desired shape, or roll out the dough with a rolling pin as thin as possible. Cut into noodles, lasagna noodles or spaghetti, or use to make ravioli.

Pasta can be cooked immediately in boiling salted water with a bit of added oil. Cooking time will vary from 1 to 4 minutes, depending on the thickness and shape of the pasta.

Uncooked pasta can be frozen in airtight bags for later use. Do not thaw frozen pasta. Cook it straight from the freezer, adding 30 seconds to 1 minute of cooking time.

*Serves 3–4*

# Old-Fashioned Strawberry Shortcake

*Spring is the best season for fresh strawberries and strawberry shortcake. Biscuits are a good choice for gluten-free baking because the crumb should be tender, not chewy. For a mixed berry shortcake, substitute a combination of blueberries, blackberries or raspberries for some of the strawberries.*

**Filling**
- 4 cups strawberries, hulled and sliced
- 3 tablespoons sugar
- Whipped Cream

**Shortcake**
- 2 tablespoons sugar
- 3 tablespoons butter, softened
- 1 egg
- ½ cup rice flour
- ⅓ cup potato starch (also known as potato starch flour)
- 2 teaspoons baking powder
- ½ teaspoon baking soda
- ½ teaspoon salt
- ¼ cup buttermilk

## Filling

Combine the strawberries and sugar in a large mixing bowl, Mix well and set aside at room temperature to blend.

## Shortcake

Preheat oven to 400 degrees and grease a baking sheet.

In a large mixing bowl, cream together the butter and sugar, then blend in the egg.

In another bowl, sift together the flours, baking powder, baking soda and salt. Add to the butter mixture in batches, alternating with the buttermilk.

Dust a work surface with rice flour and pat the dough into an 8-inch circle. Cut into 8 wedges and place on baking sheet. Bake for 12 to 15 minutes.

Split the shortcake wedges lengthwise through the middle, so each has two layers. Spoon some of the strawberry mixture onto the bottom slice, add a dollop of whipped cream and top with the top slice of shortcake. Garnish with remaining berries.

*Serves 8*

## Pizza Crust

*Pizza is one of the most popular treats for adults and kids alike. While the crust is traditionally made with wheat flour, a combination of potato starch, cornstarch, tapioca flour and powdered milk creates the right crunch, chew and color. Thinly sliced potatoes can make a hearty topping, along with cheese and fresh herbs.*

- 1 cup potato starch (also known as potato starch flour)
- ½ cup tapioca flour
- ½ cup cornstarch
- ½ cup powdered milk
- 1 tablespoon baking powder
- ½ teaspoon salt
- 2 tablespoons butter
- ¼ cup water

Preheat oven to 400 degrees. Grease 2 pizza pans.

In a large mixing bowl, mix the flours, cornstarch, powdered milk, baking powder and salt. Cut in the butter until the mixture feels like cornmeal. Pour in the water and stir until the dough forms a ball.

Knead on a lightly floured surface until smooth. Form into 2 balls.

Press each ball into a 10-inch circle on the prepared pans. Crusts should be about ¼-inch thick and edges should be ½-inch thick to contain sauce.

Top with about ½ cup of your favorite sauce and your favorite toppings. Bake for 20 to 22 minutes.

*Makes 2 crusts*

# Cupcakes

*Cupcakes have experienced a resurgence in popularity. Rice flour creates a tender crumb. Make a simple frosting by whipping together a 1-pound box of confectioners' sugar, 1 stick of butter, 1 teaspoon of vanilla and enough milk to make a spreadable consistency. You can also use a store-bought frosting (just make sure it's gluten-free), or try the Cream Cheese Frosting recipe in this book.*

- 1 cup rice flour
- 2 teaspoons baking powder
- ¼ teaspoon salt
- ½ cup sugar
- ⅓ cup butter, softened
- 1 egg
- 1 teaspoon vanilla extract
- ¾ cup milk

Preheat oven to 350 degrees. Line 12 muffin cups with paper liners.

In a medium mixing bowl, sift together the flour, baking powder and salt, and set aside.

In a large mixing bowl, cream sugar and butter with an electric mixer until light and fluffy. Beat in the egg and vanilla and mix well. Beat in milk. Stir in the flour until combined.

Spoon batter into prepared muffin cups. Transfer to the oven and bake for 20 minutes or until a cake tester or a toothpick inserted in a cupcake comes out clean.

Let cool in the pan for a few minutes before removing to a rack to cool. Frost cupcakes when completely cooled.

*Makes 12 cupcakes*

# CONCLUSION

Changing your eating habits or your entire nutritional lifestyle is never easy, and going gluten-free is no exception. If you've been directed to go gluten-free because you've been diagnosed with celiac disease or gluten sensitivity, you have quite a learning curve ahead of you. This can be daunting and overwhelming, and even make you angry at first.

As with all healthy lifestyle changes, things get easier as you adjust to new habits and new foods. That transitional time will be even easier if you can find a family member or friend with celiac disease to help you get through the process. It's essential to have someone to whom you can vent, someone who has been there and knows the issues involved. If you don't know anyone personally, consider joining a celiac support group, club or Internet forum. You may not think you'll need it, but many strong, happy people do.

Above all, keep your eye on the real goal: being safe and healthy, feeling better than you have in ages and looking forward to eating again.

Good luck, stay focused on healing, and enjoy trying new foods and new recipes.

CPSIA information can be obtained at www.ICGtesting.com
Printed in the USA
BVOW021813030413

317218BV00001B/24/P